What Others are saying about

This Is Why Your Back **HURTS**

Reading ***This Is Why Your Back Hurts*** reveals much about its author as well as his chosen topic. It reveals his intense commitment and passion in delivering compassionate chiropractic and even holistic care for his patients' spines. Multiple chapters are dedicated to tying together the contribution of anatomy, physiology, chemistry, kinetics, diet, exercise and even culture into the understanding, management, and overall well-being of our spines. ***This Is Why Your Back Hurts*** proves to be an excellent, entertaining, and even a fun read for the lay patient, trainers, and health care providers, regardless of their specialty specific roles in patient care.

—**Joseph K Jamaris MD**, *Baltimore Washington Medical Center, board certification from the member board for Neurological Surgery. Award Winner: Compassionate Doctor Recognition: 2010 & Patients' Choice Award: 2008 —2010*

It gave me a great sense of pleasure when you phoned the other day to tell me you had written a book ***This is Why Your Back Hurts.*** Here was I, an orthodox physician, who believes in Chiropractic, congratulating you for producing such a much- needed book. If only it had been in existence in the 1970's when I had numerous back patients and was suggesting to the surgeons that surgery was not the answer to most back problems. I never realized then that the answer would come from the young man I was showing round the hospital persuading him to go into Chiropractic and not Plastic Surgery. This book is an easy read and is spaced with interesting, informative anecdotes which will hold patients and doctors attention. I like the layout and presentation. A copy should be in every Medical Student Library and Chiropractic Library. Rarely, these days do we see the Whole patient considered! I received only 2 hours instruction in Supplements and Nutrition in a 5 year medical course so I was delighted with those chapters. For most of my medical life I cared for Amputees and my concerns, all the time were with Proper Human Positioning, (gait, major changes of Centre of gravity, balance etc) .Your book is timely.

—**Tony A.B. Kennard, M.D,** *Physician Orthopedic, British Health service and with Ontario Sanitarium Association, Medical Officer R.C.A.F. Aux., Amputee Coordinator with Ontario and BC Compensation Board*

Dr Vaughan Dabbs has shared with the medical community—and the world, really—what he brought back from Haiti. His time there has proven beneficial to us all for the insight he came back with.

This is Why Your Back Hurts—*Learn What You Can Do to Get Rid of the Pain* can be life changing for people who have suffered with this problem for years and I look forward to sharing it with my patients. Dabbs continues to impress me with his dedication to help people move past suffering with back pain.

—**Michael Franchetti MD**, *Johns Hopkins Howard County General Hospital, Board Certified Orthopedic & Sport Medicine Surgeon for Baltimore Raven & Washington Redskins.*

I've been raving about Dr. Dabbs since the first day I met him and his office. This book *This is Why Your Back Hurts,* is just a reminder of his dedication to help people feel better. His compassion for his patients is now available for people who do not have the luxury of having them as his doctor. This more than a good book, it is a manual to live by if you would like to never have to suffer with back pain again. This book is also unique in being the only one of its kind in addressing relevant 21st century information on the dietary and nutritional aspects for accelerating, enhancing and maintaining back health and vitality.

—**Jim Sharps, N.D., H.D., Dr.NSc., Ph.D.,** *Author of "Concepts of Original Medicine and Food & The Ideal Diet"*

I refer patients to Dr. Dabbs and they have always been happy with their patient care. This book *This is Why Your Back Hurts* is a great tribute to Dr. Dabbs dedication to helping people with back pain get on the road to recovery. This is a good book to use as a guidebook to living pain free and learning best practices. I would recommend this book to patients who would like to learn more about living back pain free!

—**Victor Kim, MD,** *Fellow of the American College of Emergency Physicians & Medical Director of AllCare of Maryland Urgent Care Centers*

This Is Why Your Back HURTS

Learn What You Can Do to
GET RID OF THE PAIN

DR. VAUGHAN DABBS

an imprint of Morgan James Publishing
NEW YORK

This Is Why Your Back **HURTS**

Learn What You Can Do to
GET RID OF THE PAIN

DR. VAUGHAN DABBS

ISBN 978-1-61448-031-0 Paperback
ISBN 978-1-61448-032-7 eBook
Library of Congress Control Number: 2011928659

Published by:

BLACK BELT PUBLISHING
an imprint of
MORGAN JAMES PUBLISHING
The Entrepreneurial Publisher
5 Penn Plaza, 23rd Floor
New York City, New York 10001
(212) 655-5470 Office
(516) 908-4496 Fax
www.MorganJamesPublishing.com

Cover Design by:
Rachel Lopez
rachel@r2cdesign.com

Interior Design by:
Bonnie Bushman
bbushman@bresnan.net

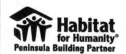

Acknowledgements

I want to thank all the people who helped me take the twenty-five year journey it took to develop this program that will enrich people's lives *one back at a time*.

I would like to thank,

My Mom and Dad who encouraged me to be a better person.

My brother Paul and sister Karen for their valuable advice.

Dr. Tony Kennard who inspired me to be a Chiropractor so I could help see those frowns turn into smiles.

Dr. Todd Johnsonbaugh for his incredible, valuable input over the last 10 years.

Joanne Colburn PT for her no problem attitude, her compassion to patient care and for all her great contributions including contributing editor, PT rehab Knowledge, and exercises instructor.

Ali Pervez, the author of " Get Your Black Belt in Marketing, www.blackbeltinmarketing.com, who directed me through the process of writing a book.

Kathryn Hayden for her modeling pictures and support for this project.

Dr. Lisa Dabbs as a contributing editor to this book and her ongoing support to make this project happen by supporting me for the last 25 years, and being a wonderful mother to our 2 sons.

My children Jesse and Austin for inspiring me to be the best that I can be so that I can show them how to be the best they can be.

Contents

Introduction
My Quest in Haiti

A Man in Search of an Answer

I am a Chiropractic Orthopedist and my passion lies in helping people with back pain. I love it when patients like Jim C. say to me, *"Wow… I can enjoy life again with my family, I can lift my kids, I can play golf, and I can live again."*

Story of Jared

It all started 22 years ago with a tragic failure that cost one man his life.

I was fresh from school, armed with theories but did not have the years of experience to back them up, when Jared came to me. He was complaining of an incessant, excruciating pain in his back from a disc herniation. I can still hear his voice clearly in my mind to this day saying… *"If you can't fix me, I swear I'll kill myself!"*

Jared had been through back surgery, he had rods of steel in his back, and the pain was still present. It was so intense that he couldn't sleep and he couldn't eat. It was simply unbearable, and I was his last resort.

I treated him seven times but he never came back for the eighth… *I failed!* I used everything I was taught in school and I did my best to help him, but it was just not good enough. I wasn't able to get rid of his pain, so he carried out his threat and he ended his own life. This shook me up…I vowed that I would never let this happen again. From that moment on I was passionate about seeking better ways of treatment.

Over the last 22 years, I researched, I talked to the best medical professionals, I attended the some of the finest seminars, and I travelled the world over in search of answers. Through these endeavors I have uncovered answers to back pain and the secrets to a healthy back. What I learned was incredible; in fact many of the things I learned were complete surprises. I am divulging these secrets to you in this book.

I know how to treat people like Jared and now have an answer for most of them. I recently have a patient Gordon T who was fused from the neck to the lower back with rods and screws from scoliosis where the spine curved like a coil.Surgeons had to use the rods and screws in order for him to function and did a good job. But he had developed pain in his lower back and could not go to work without debilitating pain. He came to me for relief saying he can't work and live like this, please help. I now have the tools to help him and after 12 weeks he is doing extremely well, working with minimal or no pain and smiling again.

My quest now in writing this book is to share my knowledge to help people like Jared and Gordon achieve a pain free life and give them a chance to live life to the fullest.

Let me tell you a little about myself, and my background. My mother was a nurse and I was simply amazed at her dedication and commitment. As far as I could remember, I knew I wanted to get into the medical/health field. When I was 16, my neighbor, a great medical doctor whom I still emulate, Dr. Tony Kennard, said to me, "Son, if I were you, I would be a Chiropractor, because people walk in with a frown and walk out with a smile." I took that to heart and went to Logan College of Chiropractic, in St. Louis, Missouri, where I became a Doctor of Chiropractic and then received a diplomat degree in Chiropractic Orthopedics from Texas Chiropractic College. It really is true what some professionals say—*when you love what to do, it never is work.*

A Surprising Find in Haiti

Recently, I went to Haiti to help people after the massive earthquake that tore their country and lives apart. I saw buildings collapsed, debris was everywhere. Destruction was a daily scene in Haiti, yet the people there were still working hard, doing what they normally did each day. I could see that even in the state they were in, they still carried on with their daily routines with smiles on their faces. Their condition never prevented them from laughing or appreciating life.

I treated hundreds of patients, young and old. In doing so, I discovered something incredible. Haitians, like people in most developing countries, have perfect and excellent posture. They stand, sit, and lie down in the right way so as to put less stress on their joints. This prevents arthritis, disc herniation, muscle spasm and many other conditions. When I treated 70, 80 and 90-year old Haitians, I was amazed to find that they had good-to-full range of motion in their spine, hips and knees. This was due to manual labor combined with good posture. Climbing up mountains with 25 pounds on their heads standing upright or doing hard manual labor with proper body mechanics ground the arthritis right out of them.

The sad fact is, we in the western culture have lost the art of **proper posture**. Proper posture means upholding the natural curve of the spine (neutral spine). This is what I call **Proper Human Positioning** or PHP which is the key to a healthy back.

Bad human positioning puts undue stress on all the joints and breaks them down before their time. Good human positioning is one of the secrets to avoiding back pain. In fact, if you truly see a Haitian standing up, it may look a little weird; to us, it's very different. Bending over, walking and running is not as we were taught, either. All of these shall be covered as we go along.

In my 22 years of practice, I've been able to treat 90% of the patients who sought my medical help in their pursuit to finally get some relief to their back pain. Posture is not what you may have been taught—having your chin up or lifting your chest up as this causes tension in the spine. We will cover the mechanics of good posture in this book, so stay tuned.

> ### *Quick Tip:*
> Test good posture by taking a picture of yourself, profile view and draw a line up from your ankle and it should pass by your ankle, hip, and shoulder and your ear. It should all line up.

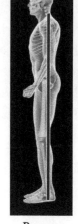

Summary:

My quest traveling to underdeveloped countries helped me discover a secret to back pain: that secret is **GOOD POSTURE** *and* **KEEPING ACTIVE**.

Proper posture— all aligned

Posture is something that used to be drilled into our heads from the time we are youngsters. But posture is often misunderstood or not taken seriously so I like to refer to it as Proper Human Postioning (PHP). Our mothers told us to stand up straight. Young girls were often made to walk back and forth across the room, stacks of books on their head, learning the basics of good posture. But those very lessons might have contributed to the waves of bad posture that are very real these days. Either we are just going too easy on the lessons that we were taught so long ago or we are just putting too much emphasis on the ramrod straight back that our mothers instilled in us. As we learned, standing too stiffly and too straight caused just as much pain and other problems as slouching ever did.

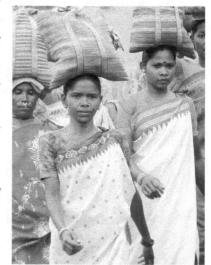

Bad posture does more than just make us look older or heavier than we are. *It does more than disappoint our mothers. As I have said, I have been able to treat the majority of people—90% in fact, who have come to me for help after being told that there was no help to be had.*

*Most of us sit in an office chair, suffering in pain even though we are doing nothing more than typing on a computer, in that cushy chair. Now, imagine if your boss told you to put a ream of paper on your head and hike it up to the top floor. You would faint! Now imagine that a woman in Haiti, twice your age is asked the same thing. She would pop that ream of paper on top of her head and get to the top floor and she would smile as she did it! The difference, we learned is not that she is stronger and she is certainly not younger—**it is all proper posture and lots of activity that allows her to do what we think of as impossible***.

1

Myths About Back Pain

Stop Believing Them!

Back pain, otherwise known as lumbago, has become very prevalent these days and there is an 80% chance you will get it over and over. Just about every person experiences backache at some point in their lives. Because of its prevalence, a lot of theories and speculations have risen regarding it. This chapter is about myths and facts surrounding back pain for the purpose of enlightening you as to what you should and shouldn't believe about it.

Walking Upright Myth

Myth: Many people believe that walking upright places more stress on your disc.

Fact: For more than 2.5 million years, we have been standing and evolution has compensated for this through proper posture and curves in the spine. So standing for millions of years on two legs has allowed a normal C curve in the back, which makes it stable.

Let's take look at four-legged creatures such as dogs or horses. I used to treat horses at the Laurel Maryland Race Track, so I've personally observed this. They have a C-curve too, which somewhat prevents their discs from bulging out.

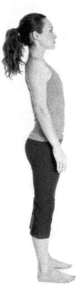

With humans, standing upright puts an S-curve in the entire back and a C-curve in the lower back. The C-curve prevents the discs from bulging. However, in developed countries, we don't have a normal smooth consistent "C" curve due to our bad posture. We sit for hours, bend, lift incorrectly, stand and walk incorrectly. Depending on your actions throughout your life, the smooth "C" curve of the lower back may be too small or too big, both of which contribute to various back problems. Due to millions of years of evolution, walking on two legs should have no more pressure on the lower back discs than walking on all fours.

Erect posture with a C curve

Age Factor Myth

Myth: The older we get the more back pains we will have.

Fact: It is a fact that we get arthritis or joint degeneration as we get older. Just like everything else, we too suffer from wear and tear. But many back problems come from disc herniations when you're in your 20s and 30s because at that age you have much more disc material to bulge out. The "jelly" inside discs dehydrates as one gets older so discs become less of a problem.

Now let's look at aging. Sure, arthritis is for older people, but it's more prevalent if you slow down, rest more, find exercising no longer appealing and, suddenly, you don't do as much manual labor anymore compared to when you were in your younger years. While it may surprise those who are not aware of the causes of back pain, this kind of sedentary lifestyle ironically causes more wear and tear on your spine. *How is this possible?* The rationale behind this fact is if you don't move, then the joints and muscles in your body will get weak due to lack of motion and activity. If you don't use it, you lose it!

In Haiti, 70-year old women carried 30-pound bags on their heads as they climbed up mountains. The old men shoveled concrete. And yet when I checked them for arthritis, they had little to none. At age 80, their knees could still bend so much that their heels touched their backside, their hips can still rotate out fully, their backs and necks still have full range of motion so that they can still twist, bend and extend fully backward. They have maintained such flexibility and sturdiness because they were forced to do manual labor, and they were exposed to physical labor their whole lives.

Manual labor grinds the scar tissues and the arthritis out of the joints, strengthens the muscles equally and continually, and develops great balance—which explains how they can still carry 30 lbs on their heads regardless of their age.

Had Haitians done physical labor with terrible posture, they would have developed back problems. Just imagine yourself carrying 30 lbs. on the back of your neck with your head down and forward. Your neck would be very sore and would build up bone spurs to stabilize itself which is *arthritis.* Picture yourself carrying 50 lbs on your back with your body flexed forward for five miles. This routine would strain your back and eventually degenerate your lower back.

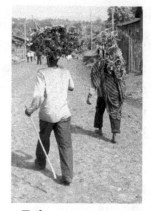

It is therefore important to maintain an active lifestyle and exercise using proper posture all day. Don't be afraid to do a little gardening or some brisk walking, house cleaning, or to move stuff here and there, and use those muscles and joints. Make this a habit and you should live life with much less back pain and arthritis.

Tribe men carrying 25 lbs on their heads have perfect posture

Height Myth

Myth: Tall people have more back problems because they have more vertebrae. In addition to this, their center of gravity is higher than the average height, which can also lead to more back problems.

Fact: Tall people have the same number of spinal vertebrae (24 total vertebras) as shorter people. They just have taller vertebrae and discs and longer muscles. This adds more support to make up for the higher center of gravity.

> ### Did You Know?
> When the Skylab Astronauts returned to Earth, it was discovered that they had grown 1.5 to 2.25 inches. The zero gravity of space had both lengthened and straightened their spines.

I have a 6'8 tall NFL football player as a patient from the Seattle Seahawks who comes in for an annual treatment of his lower back. He makes sure to get one treatment a year. That's all he needs despite the fact that he took a pounding for 15 years as an offensive center. He only needs maintenance care because he works out daily, uses perfect posture and uses proper body mechanics in everything he did in the past and presently.

The bottom line is everybody, tall or short, has an equal chance of getting back pain. The difference is in how we take care of our backs, not in our height.

> **Did You Know?**
> You are taller in the morning than you are in the evening time because of the compression of discs during our daily activity.

Weight Myth

Myth: The bigger and heavier you are, the more back problems you'll have. So, you won't be relieved of your back pain unless you lose weight.

Fact: Fifty percent of Americans overeat. Thin people have just as many back problems as fat people. The heavier or bigger a person is, the more muscles they develop in their back to help support the weight.

I had to treat a 425 lb patient named Jose B. He was a big man. It took all my strength just to lift one of his legs up. I asked him if he ever had any back problems and he said never. So I examined his spine, and I found out that he had massive back muscles. I noticed too that he had very good posture. That was the reason he never had backache even with his body mass. He had come to me for a knee issue.

A heavy person with a good posture or with a normal "C" curve in the lower back will most likely exhibit fewer back problems than a thin person with a bad posture.

Exercise Myth

Myth: The more exercise you do, the better.

Fact: Exercise is good but it has to be done in moderation. Sixty percent of Americans do not exercise. Lifting weights or doing exercises such as aerobics, yoga, and engaging in sports are good for your health. However, too much of any of these will cause overuse syndrome.

If exercising with weights it is better to lift 25% of maximum and do a lot of repetitions. It builds *endurance* that helps maintain the core back muscles, because in daily life we lift small objects such as groceries, do small tasks such as bending over to tie a shoe and other activities many times a day, not one big lift, so we need endurance more than strength.

A good example of this would be classic weight lifting. Too much of this routine will strain the body and cause the body to break down. So if you overdo exercise, your body will not recover in time.

Our body has a natural ability to heal and regenerate new tissues. However, healing doesn't come perfectly every time. When tissues are damaged, they develop scar tissues. This scar tissue is not as flexible as normal tissue. Tissues such as muscles, ligaments (they hold the bones together), tendons (they attach the muscles to the bones) and cartilage (padding between the joints) have an elastic characteristic to them. They can bounce back to their normal lengths after being stretched. Their fibers are normally paralleled and aligned, but after they're damaged and when they develop scar tissue, their fibers become crisscrossed like a spider web. Because of this arrangement, they become inflexible. Furthermore, they become less resilient and they tear and damage easily.

I had a patient, Tom B, who was in great shape. He had a ripped muscular body like a gladiator. He lifted weights daily, yet he came to see me three times a week because of pain all over his body. He didn't stop working out, so my four weeks of treatment was futile.

Later, I told him he was way over doing it and he needed to let his body recover for a day or two, and take at least four or five weeks off from the gym to undo the damage he was doing. He was reluctant, but he eventually followed my advice and his pain went away. He works out moderately now, always giving himself one or two days to recover in between workouts. He is still in great shape, and he is feeling great now.

> *Quick Tip:*
>
> The older you get, the more days rest you need to recover. Moderate exercise is needed to keep the back pain free.

Stress Myth

Myth: Stress causes back pain.

Fact: Stress can make a back problem or any illness worse, but does not in itself cause it. Stress causes tighter muscles to spasm, and this can lead to more pain. However proper posture is a relaxing posture and can lead to less stress and less back spasms. Relaxed sitting, for example, can lead to a more relaxed mental and emotional state.

I had a 25-year-old patient, Mike K., who was so stressed that when I treated him he felt better but the next day his muscles would be tight again. Exercises helped but again the next day he was so stressed he would have muscle spasms in his back again. I could not find much wrong so I asked him "What is going on with you, what are you so stressed about?" He said "I am being sued for one million dollars and its really stressing me out." I taught him proper posture and I told him to meditate for 30 minutes a day and exercise three times a week for 20 minutes full out so a desired heart rate and respiratory rate were achieved. He did these two things and he came in two weeks later all relaxed. The meditation helped his mind relax, and the intense aerobic exercises got all his frustrations out in a healthy way. I released him feeling good again.

Other Myths and Facts

Myth: Most back pain is caused by a slipped disc.

Fact: Only one to three percent of low back pain results from herniated, or slipped, discs. One of the major causes of low back pain is muscle strain from faulty posture.

Myth: Most back problems eventually require surgery.

Fact: Less than one person in 1,000 with low back pain will need surgery. Surgery is only required if major organs, such as the bladder, are affected or when mobility and sensations are greatly compromised. However, surgery is always the last option.

These days, I see surgeons only do surgery when it is absolutely necessary. The outcome is much better than 20 years ago because they do as little as possible and many use microsurgery and laser treatment. I have great respect for surgeons, for they enter the picture when everything has failed and save the day. However it is as a last resort as back surgery fails 50% of the time.

Myth: Everyone with back pain will need an MRI, and MRI is a treatment for back pain.

Fact: MRI is a diagnostic procedure; it is similar to an X-ray and CAT scan. Its purpose is to see what is really going on inside our body. In certain cases, an MRI is very useful in diagnosing back pain. However, not everyone with back pain needs this test. Try exercise, chiropractic or physical therapy first for two to four weeks and if it is not better after that, then get an MRI, CAT scan or X-ray.

Myth: Everyone has low back pain. It's something that has to be endured until it becomes disabling.

Fact: Some 6.5 million Americans are treated for low back pain each day. Getting help early is very important for successful treatment because it can resolve the problem before it worsens, and it can reduce the recurrence of the problem.

Myth: Only people who do heavy labor or a lot of lifting suffer intense low back pain.

Fact: Up to 80 percent of adults experience low back pain at some time in their lives. In addition to heavy lifting, other factors that increase the risks of developing low back pain include not having good posture, sitting for long periods without back support, driving and smoking.

Myth: Back pain will happen only once, and if it goes away it does not come back

Fact: Back pain is not an infection and we can't develop an immune response to it. Seventy percent of people with back pain that resolves will have a recurrence. Why? Oftentimes you never fixed the original cause.

> ### Did You Know?
> A disc is like jelly donut. The jelly will come out if you squeeze the donut. Same with the disc; if you squeeze it too much over time by bad posture or by an accident or by lifting wrongly, it can bulge out and burst.

Summary:

Back pain is not influenced much by the fact that we:

- *Walk on two legs*
- *Are overweight*
- *Are tall or short*

The bottom line is that we need:

- *good posture*
- *healthy diet*
- *moderate exercises*

These will go a long way to prevent and heal back problems.

Myths, especially those that have been in circulation for a long time or seem pretty reasonable **are the hardest to get rid of**. Even harder to get rid of are the myths that absolve us of any blame in the back pain that we all have from time to time. Think of this: we are among the minority when it comes to having a backbone. Of all of the creatures on the planet, 97% of them have no backbone at all and yet 90% of the people in the developed world will have some form of back pain during their lifetime.

We have this back pain **because we do not have good posture and because we are confused about exercise**. We have an all-or-nothing-at-all attitude about exercise—we are either doing too much exercise or not enough. Either we are working out too strenuously or we are not working out hard enough. We think that if we are tall and fit and thin that we will never have a problem with our back at all and then we get out there and overdo it. Remember the story about the ripped patient (Tom B.)? He continued to have pain even after four weeks of treatment simply because he was not willing to give up his daily workouts. He was simply overdoing it. Once he allowed himself the time to let his body rest and recover, when he started approaching exercise with a more moderate approach, he was able to be pain free.

From the long, stretched neck of the giraffe to the tiny little mouse, we all have the same number of vertebrae with which to work with. Allowing ourselves to be lazy about our posture gives us the problems that we want to blame on other things: we hate our beds, it's our height, our weight, a combination of all the above. But those are all myths. The truth is simple: **we need to work on our posture and exercise key areas and most of our back pain will be a thing of the past**.

2
Back to Basics

The Back, It's Basic Structure, How It Works

A mechanic needs to know an engine before he can fix it—before you heal your back you must understand how it works. My patient Bob M., a car mechanic, said to me *"Why do I need to know how my back works? I'm in pain and I want to be out of pain—that's all."* I said to him *"Bob, how can you fix the engine on your own car if you don't know how the engine works?"* He got the analogy. I continued *"With a car, you can hire a mechanic such as yourself to fix it by replacing the defective parts, but in your back there are no spare parts, so only you can take care of it."* Bob now understood. So understand how your back works, then you will know how to take care of it. Most people take better care of their car than their back. They get oil changes and tune ups, wash it, clean it. It's time to learn about your back so you can get it tuned up.

Anatomy of Your Back

Your back is made up of bones, joints, muscles and cartilage or *discs*. There are 24 movable blocks called vertebrae (bones) in your entire spine, including five in the lower back, and in between each of these blocks is a piece of cartilage type of material called a disc, which is tough on the outer layers and jelly-like in the middle. Each vertebra has two joints called *facets* that stop the vertebrae from twisting too far.

17

The spine contains the spinal cord, which transmits nerve stimuli from the brain and sends them simultaneously everywhere in the body. These nerves go to the body's vital organs including the intestines and bladder, to the muscles then to the skin. All sensations are pretty much covered by the nervous system. It stands to reason a structurally sound spine with nerves traveling out to the rest of the body is a healthy spine. The nervous system extends through a healthy body like a garden hose watering plants; if there is a kink in the hose, less water is produced thus the flowers wither.

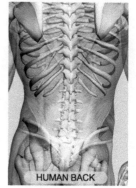

HUMAN BACK

Human back

In the lower back, there are the deep muscles called the **Multifidi** and Erector Spinae. These muscles help stabilize and move the individual vertebrae. There are also other stabilizer muscles called the *core* muscles—mainly the abdominal muscles over the belly and pelvic muscles. These muscles act like guide wires on a tower.

Your Back is Like a Radio Tower

Using this analogy with a tower, you will be able to clearly understand the structure of the back. The tower stands straight up on solid ground; the wires are equally tight on either side and tied all around.

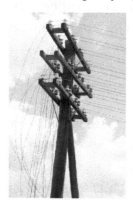

Tower and guide wires

If the tower starts to blow one-way or the other, the wires hold it in place. If there is no wind, the strong metal frame in the tower holds itself up. But if the base or ground starts to sink or give way on one side, or there is lots of wind, the tower will lean. The support wires on the side the tower leans toward become loose. The other side of the tower the support wires get overly tight and start to tear. The metal in the tower will get overly stressed and then eventually bend or crumble.

So with Proper Human Positioning (PHP) your lower back acts similarly to a radio tower held up by wires. It has a natural C curve of stacked vertebrae (the metal tower) that is stabilized by the *multifidi* muscles (the support wires) in the back and core muscles or the pelvic and abdominal muscles in the front (the stable ground at the base of the tower).

The C curve works best because it functions like a spring for jumping and moving. The base is your pelvis, which rocks back and forth but when stationary, it sits tilted forward so that the belt buckle in the front is slightly below the back of the belt, which we call the **anteriopelvis**. This part is vital to balance the backward "C" in your lower lumbar spine. If that base or pelvis shifts too far forward or backward, that causes strain on the spine. The muscles will then wear out, collapse or waste away on one side and become spasmed or tight on the other.

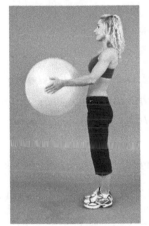

Good posture—see the c-curve in the lower back

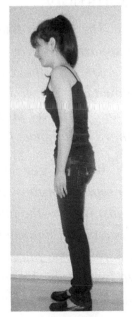

Bad posture showing a posterior pelvis

I had a patient Dan H. who had good-looking posture to most who see him, but to me he had very little lumbar curve. This was due to his pelvis rotating back (retropelvis or posterior tilted pelvis) and flattening out his spine. I asked him, "Ever had back problems?" He pulled up his shirt and showed me scars in his lower back from two back surgeries. A posterior tilted pelvis makes the disc more susceptible to disc herniation.

A normal pelvis or base with good spine posture gives us a relaxed pelvic muscle, which allows a normal bladder and intestinal flow. A posterior or too anterior pelvis or one that is rotated too far back or forward, disrupts this muscle structure and can cause inconsistencies, cystitis, prostititis and pelvic floor myalgia as well as birth difficulties, pain in the back, hip and arthritis.

A properly structured spine that is cared for through proper posture at work, rest or play and exercised is like a well-maintained car. It will last longer and you will be healthier and pain free.

I had an 85-year-old woman with really good posture come in for a sprained wrist. I asked her *"have you had any back, neck or other organ problems?"* She responded *"No, why?"* I said, *"Because you have really good posture and that usually promotes a healthy spine and organs."* She just smiled and said *"well I was taught as a child to stand up straight and I watched my parents, who also had perfect posture and good health."*

We in this culture seem to have lost that art—hence all the back, hip and knee pain, arthritis and other problems such as prostititis, bladder issues and birth difficulties.

Summary:

*The **spine is like a radio tower** and needs to be **supported by strong support wires** to be able to withstand stresses of gravity and other stressors. Weakness in these wires will cause **instability** and the tower will break down fast. Our lower backs are shaped a certain way and disrupting that shape with bad posture will cause it to break down fast, like a car tire that's misaligned. Only we can't replace your spine like we can a tire.*

We only get one spine and while medical science has found ways to replace organs and parts of the human body, there is no mechanical substitute for the human spine. The spine comprises of 120 muscles, 220 specialized ligaments and over 100 joints. When we are born, we have 33 vertebrae but by the time we reach adulthood, that number is down to twenty-six. The other nine bones are fused: four of them become the tailbone and five become the back of the pelvis.

***There is no changing the basics of the spine**—it is the same for the old and the young, the thick and the thin, the active and the couch potato.*

With the exception of a few rare, medical cases, there are no differences in one spine to the next, physically that is. How that person uses that spine is the issue. Learning how posture affects our back health is important but it is equally important to have a basic understanding of how the spine works. Like I said before, we know more about the car that we drive, and we take better care of it than we do our spines.

*We need to **be sure that we are doing everything that we can to learn** what can possibly be wrong with our back and how best to care for it. We need to understand how deeply a back problem **can affect our entire lives,** not just because of the pain that we feel but because of the stress and worries that the pain may bring.*

Something to think about*: People who have an initial issue with back pain and do not retrain their deep back muscles are up to twenty two times more likely to have a recurrence of that back pain within the following three years.*

3

The Real Causes of Back Pain—*What Most Doctors Won't Tell You*

Back Pain: A Worldwide Language

The causes of back pain are nearly as numerous as terms used to describe the symptoms. Back pain is a primary reason people seek medical attention. Bearing in mind that almost 80% of the adult population will have some form of back pain, it could be said that back pain is a universal outbreak or epidemic. Back pain recognizes no age, gender or ethnic barriers, but pain does indicate there is a problem, and we need to find out what is causing it. So we begin testing.

> **Did You Know?**
> There is a 6% – 10% chance that one back pain episode may become a long-term disability. Outcomes are 10 times worse if pain is radiating down the leg.

The Various Causes of Back Pain

Some of the major causes of back pain are:

- Bad posture that includes unbalanced weak or tight muscles and joints

- Accidents such as auto accidents or sports injuries

- Genetically weak discs or cartilage

- Compression fractures from osteoporosis

- Arthritis of the back and spine due to wear and tear

- Pathologies such as cancer, psoriasis, rheumatoid arthritis, and many others

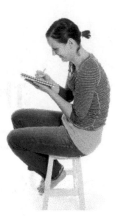

Bad posture

Understanding Proper Human Positioning or Posture and Its Relation to Back Pain

Posture is too light a word, but I prefer the term *Proper Human Positioning* because posture can be taught many different ways but realy there is only one way that's the best for the body to be in it's lowest energy form and stable known as the "proper human position". When we think of posture we think stand up straight like a military man or women but that uses far too much energy and places far too much stress on the muscle in your back. But for simplicity I will use the word posture but realize I'm realy talking about perfect human positioning in all situations from standing to sitting to bending to sleeping.

What is not well taught or understood in all the medical fields is that most back problems stem from bad posture. Those who sit, stand, walk or lift incorrectly with faulty body mechanics dramatically increase their odds of suffering back pain. Sport injuries, arthritis, weak discs and accidents will all have worse outcomes if the back is already compromised by bad posture.

If your car hits a pothole and a tire misaligns, then it wears out many times faster. The car will pull to one side and eventually the tire will blow all due to being misaligned. This is similar with the spine.

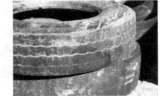

Back pain was not common until the 20th century. We used to have good posture prior to this time. Posture in its best form was taught from generation to generation. But in the 1920s it was fashionable to slump, and that was the end of generations of good posture.

A misaligned tire wears out fast, just like bad posture and your spine wearing out

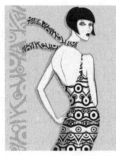

In 1950, however, back pain was twice as common. People thrust their pelvis and necks forward and hunched their shoulder as a fashion statement. That was the death of the proper posture culture. We've been using computers, sitting on couches watching TV, lifting incorrectly for the last 90 years, and that's not enough time for the spine to develop changes to support these postural issues so it breaks down.

It was fashionable to slump

By contrast, many people in traditional cultures in Africa, Haiti and parts of Asia and other developing cultures still retain proper posture deep in their culture and thus only 5-10% of these populations suffer from back pain versus 80% in western culture. When I visited these developing countries and observed those cultures, I saw them do heavy manual labor such as bending all day in rice fields, or carrying blocks of concrete on their heads. They hardly ever complained of back problems because they did it with correct posture.

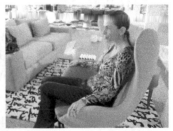

Bad posture in the 1920's started with chairs that forced bad posture like this

So, what are we really talking about here? We are talking about the poor posture that is the basis of most back pain. Posture is held by *core* and *multifidi* muscles. How we stand, sit, lie down, walk, bend and lift should be taught in all cultures; however in western society it is not. We've been inclined to somehow take that for granted. We slouch, walk by forcing our legs forward, work with computers or at a desk all day, watch TV for hours on a comfortable couch that has little support. We do everything in flexion—even work out with weights or aerobics in flexion (thrusts forward). We hardly ever work out the mid back, lower back, hamstrings, gluteus medius, hip muscles (abductors and adductors). We work out the front body muscle—the *pectoralis, anterior deltoids, quadriceps*—which gives us that forward body tilt and too much pelvic tilt, and later that hump in the mid back like the Hunchback of Notre Dame we all dread. This happens just from normal activity such as sitting at a computer all day hunched over or sitting on a couch that forces your spine to slump.

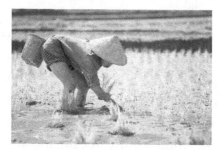

A women working in the rice field-pay special attention to how she bends at her hip and knees

What Is Proper Human Positioning or Posture?

Proper human positioning or posture is a lost art, but still very prevalent in tribes in Africa, Asian farming communities, Haitians and other developing countries where it is their culture to stand, sit erect and bend not at the back but at the hips. In ancient times, during the primeval years of man, we used to spend 12 hours a day hunting, gathering and being active. Now we sit in chairs in front of computers and our television sets.

Proper posture entails retaining the natural curve of the spine called neutral spine. Not only should proper posture be used when standing or sitting, but also it should be included into all activities of daily living—thus minimizing the amount of harmful stress the spine must bear. Standing up too straight as we were taught causes the spine to arch and compress and also causes back pain injury. Slumping places too much pressure on the discs of the lower back and they can bulge out and herniate, pinching nerves—ouch!

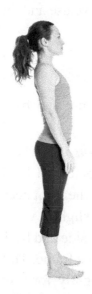

Good posture- notice hips over knees, over the ankles, shoulders are back, head back, chin slightly down

Going to the gym three times a week is good but not necessary if you practice good posture and change your daily activities so you walk more. Try parking further away and walking to work, climbing steps instead of taking an elevator, doing squats at work etc.

Let's look at a posture of a typical Haitian. They stand erect. The head is back but not too far back, the ear is over their shoulders and the chin is slightly down. Their shoulders are far back and down. The pelvis is rotated forward so as to give a C curve to the lower back. You need a consistent C from L1-S1 or upper low back to the sacrum. Anyone, big or small, can learn to maintain this posture.

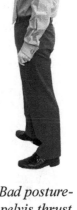

Bad posture- pelvis thrust forward, head too far forward

Notice that their hips are directly above their knees which are above their ankles. Their knees are straight up and down and slightly bent and not turned in but slightly outward. The pelvis has a lot to do with this.

They have good arches in their feet, as they walk heel first and that arch rotates the hips far forward. This is an indicator that the person has a healthy posture.

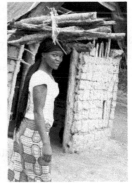

Typical haitian with perfect posture being active

This excellent overall posture Haitians and other developing countries have and were taught culturally gives them only a five percent chance of back pain versus the western society with its bad posture and 80% chance of back pain in their lives. It's a major issue to solving the cause and preventing back pain, so let's look at the different postures we use and the problems that stem from them.

What Muscles are Involved in Good Posture?

Weak muscles or overly tight muscles cause bad posture and back pain. The key muscles are the following:

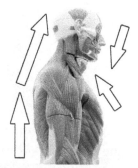

Force direction where the chin tilts down stretching the back of the neck and elongating the entire spine

Neck Flexors and Extensors: These are very important to the spine and back because the flexors which are the front neck muscles pull the head down slightly while the extensors which are at the side and back of the neck hold the head on the frame. This balance act has the head slightly forward chin slightly down so the head pulls on the spine elongating it. This forces antigravity on the spine which helps prevent slow degeneration or arthritis. If the neck is not positioned correctly then the low back and spine will be thrown off balance.

Multifidi Muscles: When you mention the multifidi muscles, most doctors will go multifidi what? These are very misunderstood and unacknowledged muscles yet eighty percent of people suffering from back pain have weak or atrophied (wasted away) multifidi muscles. These are the muscles that run up and down your back right beside the spinous processes or the bumps in the center of your back. They run from

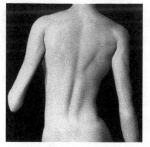

Muscles protruding either side of the spine are the key stabilizers called the mulifidi muscles

the sacrum to the base of the skull. They hold up, lengthen and support the spine. They are the key stabilizers of the spine.

Within 24 hours of a back injury such as lifting a box incorrectly, sleeping twisted or having a car accident, one can injure a single joint and the surrounding multifidi muscles will lose size by 25%. This leads to instability, which leads to many other bad things such as disc herniation, arthritis, etc. If one side is atrophied, the vertebrae will shift and become unstable. It's like a car's tire that was misaligned; the tire and vertebrae will wear out and the tire or disc will blow out.

Core Muscles: In addition to the weak multifidi muscles, weak core muscles play a major role in back pain. Core muscle support the pelvis and lower back. These are mainly the abdominal and pelvic muscles (mainly the Psoas muscle). If you have weakness here, the posture collapses.

The Abdominal Muscles which are the Abdominal Erectus and Transverse muscles are at the front and sides of the belly and just like the multifidi muscles which help the spine from falling forward these help in preventing the spine from falling backward.

The Psoas Muscles which are found deep in the back, connects the lumbar spine to the pelvis. This muscle plays a key role in supporting the

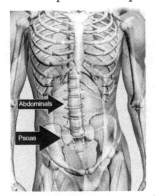

spine in relation to the pelvis and it helps with elastic support to hold up and stabilize the spine. It also influences the diaphragm for breathing. Quite often, this muscle is too tight. One can feel pain in the groin or lower abdominal quadrant when this muscle is in spasm.

Too many abdominal sit ups or leg raises or sitting all day or walking the way most of us do shortens and tenses this muscle. It needs to be relaxed and elastic to allow free movement of the hip, legs, spine and diaphragm. Proper

Abdominals and psoas are key core stabilizers

posture as one can see, allows proper breathing and less tension and a relaxed, pain free body.

Hamstrings: These long muscles are found at the back of the thigh and often get too short in westerners who are sitting all day and night. These, along with the Gluteus muscles maintain the proper extension of the pelvis and flexion of the knees. The hamstrings, if too short or tight cause the pelvis to shift posteriorly, which can put a lot of stress on the lumbar discs.

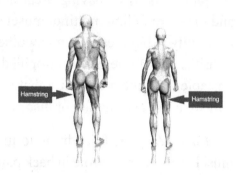

The Feet: They are the base of the entire structure. To have a healthy base is a great start. But many of us walk in shoes that have too much support and this doesn't allow the foot muscles to work naturally. Restrictive shoes such as high heels distort the feet and cause them to lose the arch. This will cause bunions and plantar fasciitis, and continue the destruction up the body.

Posture, Strength and Flexibility

A common misunderstanding is that our muscles must be strong to support us, but in fact the opposite is true. Muscles must be supple and elastic and able to withstand 25% of full strength for a long period of time and not 100 % strength for short periods. Muscles that are too strong or too tense, as many of us have, compress the misaligned joints and break them down, causing arthritis.

Overdeveloped flexor muscles such as the chest muscle (pectorals), front thigh (quadriceps), and front hip area (psoas muscles) pull the body forward into flexion. In addition to this, tight back of the thigh muscles (hamstrings) pull the pelvis back reducing the C curve and opening the discs up in the back, which puts enormous pressure on them to blow out.

What causes all this?

Sitting all day in flexion shortens the hamstrings and puts the body on flexion. Working out at the gym lifting flexion weights (such as bench press, lifting squats, bicep curls) or aerobics (such as stair steppers and many other machines) overwork the flexors, as does hard labor where you lift with your back and not your hips. It's hard to escape working in flexion but no worries; we will cover how to avoid this later in the book. But here is a picture below of the wrong way and the right way to sit as one example:

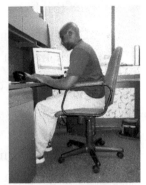

Wrong way to sit—see he is bent forward

My patient John T. was 40 years old and had low back, mid back, and neck pain for months especially after a long days work at a desk. When I looked at his posture, he looked like an 80 year old, with a hump in his back. We worked with him to straighten him out through spinal manipulation, strengthening and stretching his key muscles and reworking his ergonomic station at work until he exhibited good posture mechanics every day and straightened out. His pain left and he gained a couple of inches in height. He looked like he was healthy and he was.

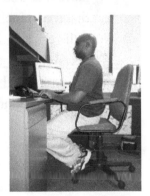

Right way to sit— see his legs are under the chair and forces him to lean back and take the stress off the low back muscles and disc.

Three Types of Wrong Posture

1. **Anteverted pelvis**—This is a forward pelvis with the spine leaning back known as lumbar *hyperlordosis*–Remember the "C" curve that I mentioned before in the lower back? In this type of posture, the letter "C" is exaggerated or there is too big a curve at the lower back area.

This type of posture causes:

- Tightening of the muscles in the lower back and the hamstring muscles at the back of the thighs.

- Overdevelopment of the quadriceps muscles at the front of the thighs.

- The stomach to stick out

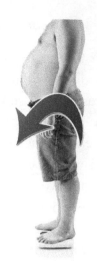

- Approximation of the facet joints on the back of each set of vertebrae. The facet joints of the vertebrae form tunnels for the nerves to pass through from the spine. When the spine has too much of a curve, these tunnels become narrow and sometimes they become so narrow that they pinch on the nerves, which of course will result in intense pain. Also, because the vertebrae are too near each other, excessive friction is inevitable. As a result, there will be wear and tear that will eventually lead to a form of arthritis called spondylosis. Bottom line…still pain!

Lumbar hyperlordois due to front of pelvis too far forward

I have a 50-year-old patient named Melody H. who used to be a gymnast as a teenager. She puts her lower back into hyperextension all the time. She has a swayback posture that is characterized by the pelvis being too far forward. She looks like she's leaning back all day long. This faulty posture caused unnecessary pressure on her lower back facet joints, which caused them to degenerate into bad arthritis and lots of pain.

2. **Retroverted pelvis**—This is the backward pelvic tilt and leaning forward body or lumbar hypolordosis. This flattens the lower back C-curve, which causes:

- Little support for the spine

- Overdeveloped upper trapezius neck muscles

- Compressed lung capacity

- Disc bulging or herniation
- Tight hamstrings

A proper pelvis rotates forward causing a C-curve in the lower back. When you lie on your back, put your hand under the lower back curve to feel this C. The retropelvis posture causes flattening

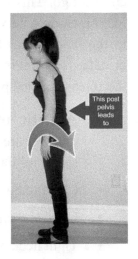

or *hypolordosis* of the lumbar C curve. This places far too much pressure on the lower two discs (L4-L5 and L5-S1) of the spine and can cause those discs to bulge or be herniated backward and

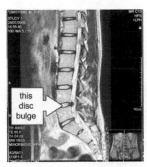

A pelvis rotated too far back causing hypolordosis or flattening of the spine leading to disc bulges

pinch nerves. A normal lumbar spine C-curve contains the discs so they don't bulge backward onto the spinal cord or onto the nerves that exit the spine.

Reducing this C pushes the jelly in the middle of that disc back through the tougher exterior cartilage and it can bulge on the outer layers and onto the nerves or blow out completely. This adds pressure and pinches off the nerve. This then leads to pain, muscle spasm and weakness along the leg or pain or numbness down one or both legs. If it's the nerve to your foot muscles that gets pinched off, it can give your foot a weakness often known as the "foot drop". Every step you take may cause your foot to flop to one side.

If it's the bladder nerve that's pinched *(cauda equana syndrome)*, it can prevent you from urinating, thus causing your bladder to accumulate waste. This case would call for emergency surgery.

I had a patient Ken F. who came in with severe back pain radiating down his leg to his foot. But that was not the worst of his problems. He also complained of not being able to go to the bathroom and urinate. Nothing would come out yet he felt he had a full bladder and was frustrated he couldn't go. This was an emergency because the disc in his back was not just pinching a nerve root; it was pinching the spinal cord and the nerves to the bladder. So the bladder's valves would not release to be able to urinate. He went into surgery to remove the herniated disc that night and the release of that pressure allowed him to urinate again.

3. **Athletic or Military Posture**–This is where all the back muscles are used to stand as tall and erect as possible, which you see in military for example. It causes:

- Chest to be lifted reducing lung capacity
- Head and chin back causing excess strain on the neck
- Tight neck muscle and spine causing constant tension and the urge to stretch
- Early arthritis from the excessive strain

This posture is seen in military personnel and weight lifters and is due to over working the back extensor muscles. It looks good, and many people mistake it for great posture, but if you tried to stand absolutely upright and tall as possible it would look like this. Try it, how does it feel? You should feel all the muscles in your back engaged and if you kept this up all day long every day those muscles would wear out and develop knots, which are painful and radiate constant pain and a sensation of needing to stretch. These tight muscles would put undue stress on the back joints leading to early arthritis or disc bulges.

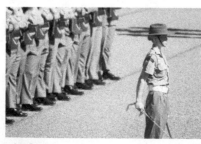

Military posture uses too many muscles and stiffens them

I had a patient, Sergeant Efrem M, who had pain all over. The army could not do anything for him and he was frustrated and wanted to quit. His posture was to stand in a military stance, completely upright with head held high and leaning back slightly. He looked good, as all military men and women do at attention, but this posture was compressing the joints in his back all day long. We treated him with manipulation, exercise to loosen up muscles, and posture training. He quickly got better and remained in the military, pain free.

What Does Proper Posture Look Like?

Standing Proper Posture:

- The pelvis should be tipped slightly forward or *anteverted* so that the belt line is slightly lower in the front than the back.

- The forward pelvic tilt causes a C-curve in the lower back with the angle in the lower two vertebrae should be a little less than the angle in the upper lumbar spine.

- The shoulders should be positioned backward in relation to the torso. The arms should be externally or outwardly rotated so the palms are facing forward. Most westerners who spend long working hours with computers or westerners who are engaged in weight lifting carry their shoulders forward and this places undue stress on tendons and ligaments of the shoulders causing tendonitis, bursitis, capsulitis and other kinds of inflammation.

- The neck angle is seen by the chin angle. The chin should be angled slightly downward so the cervical spine (the segment of the spine in the neck area) is elongated.

- The buttocks should be well developed for walking and running. Most westerners use their quadriceps or thigh muscles instead of their buttocks in walking or running. This will affect the hip, knees and feet and will cause a myriad of problems. You need to use the buttocks—the gluteal muscles and back of the thigh-hamstring muscles—to walk and run, and not the front thigh-quadriceps muscles. You will learn more about this later in the book in Chapter 7.

- There should be a groove running along the spine that shouldn't be too deep and should not show the prominence of the vertebrae.

- The rib cage should be full and should hang from the spine and the sternum or the breastbone. The top part of the rib cage should be raised, but the lower part should be level with the abdominal area. This will give more volume to each breath, which will lead to greater lung capacity, more oxygen and more energy. Most of us in western culture have diminished lung capacity.

- The hips should be parked straight over the knees. Westerners usually have their hips forward. This faulty posture places more pressure on the hip joint, leading to more bone-to-bone friction and arthritis, tendonitis and bursitis. Forward misalignment of the hips also places a lot of pressure on the veins, arteries and nerves that travel from the spine down to the legs causing nerve problems that may result in cold feet, Reynaud's syndrome and slower healing of leg injuries, especially among diabetics.

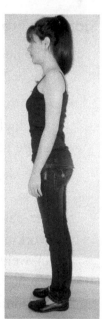

- The knees should be slightly bent and not locked into place and should point straight or slightly outward. "Knock-knees" are common among westerners and these cause knee ligament and cartilage tearing, and make the knees prone to arthritis.

Image of a good standing posture

- The feet should have arches and most of the weight should be placed on the heel because it is reinforced. The front of the foot is delicate and cannot support full body weight for long periods of time. In our culture, many women wear high heeled shoes, which put a lot of weight on the forefoot causing a lot of foot problems such as bunions, neuritis, plantar fasciitis and many other conditions including back pain.

Posture Training

Very little proper posture training is done. Good posture is a lifestyle change and takes practice. It's not a quick fix. But really there is no quick fix. Back pain usually takes months to years of destructive forces to develop in the lower back. Bad posture is the most common of these destructive forces. Fix the posture and the muscles, joints, tendons and ligaments—the building blocks needed to support the spine—all become healthier and stronger. Just a few weeks of conscious training will help your posture and prevent or reverse most back problems.

Practice and put reminders or triggers such as sticky notes at work and in every room at home, set up your chairs, bed, etc. to be posture friendly. Do it for your health. Practice by walking and sitting with a book on your head; try it daily for a week and feel what good posture is like. See Chapter 6 for how to get and practice proper posture.

Useful Tips:

The feet are the support base for the rest of the body. If you lose your support arch, you lose the support for your spine. Do foot exercises to help rebuild your arch and presto, you will see the bunion go away, and your pelvis will sit in its proper place. Your back pain may go away.

To exercise the foot, try to walk barefoot whenever possible, as this will work all the muscles in the foot and add flexibility.

To exercise the foot for arch restoration:

Stand with feet six inches apart

Step 1: Lift your right heel off the floor slightly

Step 2: Turn the right foot toes slightly left or inward

Step 3: Hold the floor with your toes and the ball of your forefoot and bring the heel in toward the center of the body line, the knees will roll right away from the center

Step 4: Bring the heel to the floor and put weight on the outside of the foot. You will feel you have an arch now. Repeat on left foot

Do this daily and hold for as long as you can on both feet. If wearing shoes, try this with the shoes on but it may be difficult so concentrate on turning the knees away from each other and straighten them, but do not lock them. Orthotics can help also, but you still need to exercise the foot without shoes.

Summary:

Proper posture looks different from what we're used to seeing. **It is crucial to learn and practice proper posture to eliminate back issues,** *such as disc herniations and arthritis. It all starts with the structure of the pelvis, which is influenced by your feet and how you stand, lie or sit daily.* **Those with proper posture like most in developing countries have only a five to ten percent chance of back pain versus an 80 percent chance for those in the western developed world.** *Bad posture is by far the number one cause of back pain. Practice proper posture and your chances of back pain will go down substantially. In fact, hip, knee and foot problems will also diminish greatly as well!*

Spinal disorders are number one on the list of causes for disability *in the working, adult population and the number two reason for doctor visits. And while it is usually considered to be the last resort, spinal problems are the third most common reason for all surgeries. Think about it: we start a new job, we get a new chair. After a few days, we notice that our back is hurting. We take some pain medications and then we go about our daily routine, making no adjustments whatsoever. The pain might go away* *on days when we are not at work but will certainly come back when we go back to that new office. Finally, we go to the doctor who starts treatments that may mask a few of the symptoms but will not address the actual problem. We go on and on until we are sitting in the surgeon's office.*

Our lack of proper posture in this culture has led us to not only increased pain in the back but a lack of proper breathing as well. Unfortunately, we are also a culture that values the quick fix. ***Proper posture training takes practice;*** *it takes effort and concentration. It is about making a change for your entire life, a change that is as important as choosing healthy foods and moderate exercise.*

4

What Went Wrong?

Different Types of Back Problems and Available Treatments

Coccydynia: The coccyx is the end point of the spine; it is usually called the tailbone.

Coccydynia is a condition wherein sitting causes soreness in the tailbone area. You can get this from trauma or from falling square on the buttocks. It can cause a perianal cyst, which is an infected boil on the tailbone area. This condition can last for years. Deep tissue massage can help with the trauma. Antibiotics are necessary if it is caused by an infected cyst.

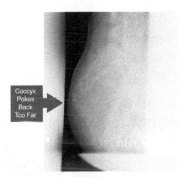

Coccyx or tailbone on X-ray

Disc Bulges and Herniations

So what does this bad posture, weak multifidi and core muscles, tight hamstrings and psoas muscle, cause in the end?—It causes a myriad of problems, one of which is a disc bulge or herniation.

The discs between the two lowest spinal vertebrae are highly susceptible to bulging backward and when this happens, the jelly in the middle will eventually squirt out, or herniate, and sit right on a nerve or the spinal cord. When this disc bulges or herniates, it can pinch the nerve root that exits from the back of the spine and goes down the leg and the foot. This can cause radiating pain, hypersensitivity or numbness along the length of the impinged nerve.

Upon physical examination, there will be a decreased tendon reflex (reflex hammer test) when there's an impingement and a relative leg or foot muscle weakness. Having two out of three of these signs is considered an indication that back surgery is necessary.

However, keep in mind that most of the time it's not the bulging disc or herniated disc that causes pain in the back and down the leg to the foot. Often times, it's the inflammation or swelling of the nerves from too much stretch from faulty posture that causes it. Eliminate that and the disc poses no problem. Half of the over 50 population has disc bulges or herniations, and they usually never know it.

Beware of results of tests such as the MRI, CAT scan or X-ray. These tests can be amazing to help a doctor to see what is going on in the spine. Although MRIs, X-rays, CAT scans show great images, they don't really correlate to the problem. It may show a disc bulge and the person has no pain, or it might be normal yet the person is in pain. An MRI, CAT scan or X-ray show static pictures only and most back problems are due to moving mechanical dysfunctions, like a car tire being misaligned. A spine is a moving, living object. An MRI, CAT scan or X-ray will be like me taking a picture of a tire in the driveway standing still; it won't show the misalignment. But if you took a movie of the tire on the highway going 60 mph, you could see it wobbling. This can be noticed in the spine with a motion X-ray and this is a valuable tool to show this dysfunctional movement. A static MRI, X-ray or CAT scan will not show this.

I published an article in SPINE JOURNAL about X-ray results showing very little about a person's pain. My study found that X-rays don't really correlate to a person's back problems. Therefore, don't rely too much on the results of your diagnostic exams because they are not sure indications of your prognosis. They are a tool or a small piece of the puzzle.

I had a patient Michelle M. who had a huge disc herniation on an MRI and had burning spasms in her back mostly at the end of a workday. She had painful epidural injections and PT traction. This treatment only made her condition worse. We relaxed the muscles with massage and found out that her posture at work bending forward at her desk fatigued the muscles, and that caused the burning. We corrected for this with use of a Swedish kneeling chair and taught her proper posture and her back pain disappeared. The lesson here was the disc shown on MRI was not relative to her problem.

Some doctors tend to place too much emphasis on the MRI when it is only a small piece of the puzzle. However, there are a few instances where MRI will help if all the history, all the other exam findings and tests point to the same thing. This is rarer than you think. To really find what's going on, you need an arsenal of tests such as a good history taking, posture analysis, a full orthopedic, neurological and physical exam. You don't need a full blood test unless your symptoms are unusual for back pain or they are not going away with proper care.

My patient Michelle M. would not have had her back pain go away, and would have most likely had more painful epidurals and surgery if we had not taken a full history and analyzed her posture. If the MRI shows up disc herniation, the exam shows up disc herniation, and her history correlates to that, then these methods would have worked.

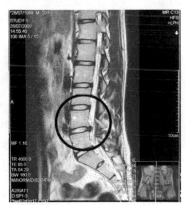

MRI *shows disc herniation*

An MRI, CAT scan or X-ray is not necessary right away. A good history and orthopedic and neurological exam can figure out 90% of most back problems. A chiropractor, physical therapist or medical doctor can do these. If the patient then undergoes treatment for the problem and it fails to respond in two to four weeks, then it may be necessary to take MRIs and X-rays.

Certain neurologic symptoms may indicate the need for immediate medical attention and need an MRI and other image tests immediately. These 'red flags' include bowel or bladder dysfunction, extremity weakness or numbness.

I saw a patient Mark M who had a disc herniation the size of my thumb on an MRI. His herniation was huge and it squeezed far into the spinal cord. You might think that is was a surgical emergency, but he was symptom free after two weeks of treatment. On the other hand, I had another patient George S. who had no findings on his MRI but he had pain for weeks that would not go away. Tests and findings don't always tell you who you will heal.

Facet Syndrome

The facets are where the two joints in the back of each two vertebrae lock and prevent someone from turning too much. This interlocking produces a lot of friction within the joints that wears out the thin cartilage between them. As a result, spurs develop or swelling and inflammation occur. The pain experienced here is usually radiating pain. Sometimes the pain radiates or shoots down to the mid thigh. This condition can be best managed with rehab exercises and chiropractic manipulation. This diagnosis is underutilized but many people suffer from it. If you have lower back pain that radiates only to the knee and no further, you have a high probability of having facet syndrome.

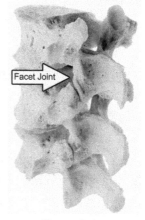

Facet Joint

Facet joint

I have had many patients come in with this condition and who almost immediately felt better after just one chiropractic adjustment or manipulation.

Muscle Spasm

This is rarely a cause of back pain but is a result of another back problem. This is just a protective mechanism of the body to prevent more injury. When there is muscle spasm, you can be absolutely sure that there is an injury somewhere. This is a very common misdiagnosis. The diagnosis should not be reliant on the premise that a patient has a mere muscle spasm and only needs a muscle relaxer. The diagnosis should be based on what is exactly causing the spasm. Always look for the cause. Otherwise, you'll just be chasing the symptoms. In rehab, chiropractic manipulation works well in targeting the root causes of such spasms, which are usually associated with posture, injury or joint dysfunction in the spine due to wear and tear.

Muscle relaxers are good for short-term relief, but they cannot get rid of the real problem.

Osteoarthritis

This is one kind of arthritis that results from the natural wear and tear of our joints. It is also known as DJD (degenerative joint disease). When osteoarthritis happens in the joints of the spine, the condition is called *spondylosis* In this condition, the spaces through which the nerves pass as they branch out from the spinal cord, narrows down. Spondylosis is often accompanied by impinged nerves. Furthermore, as the bones start to regenerate bone spurs develop all around the vertebrae causing more impingements.

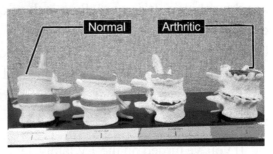

4 stages of spinal degeneration from left to right -stage 1 normal. stage 2 – thinning disc. stage 3 thin disc, bone spurs developing stage 4-fused spine

I have seen arthritis in 30 year olds, especially after traumas such as car accidents. However, it doesn't have to be this way. I have seen

90 year olds with very little or no arthritis. I treated many Haitians with great posture who were 70-90 with little or no arthritis and great ranges of motion. Genetics can play a factor and so can traumas. However, proper exercise, rehabilitation after injury and execution of proper posture go a long way in preventing this. In some cases, the pain and discomfort are reversed and not felt again.

I had a patient named Mary S, and she was 92 years old. She had giant spurs in her back, thin discs and yet good posture. She always exercised and her range of motion was good. She came in for shoulder pain, not back pain. Pretty impressive for her age!

Osteoporosis

Do you ever see older people that are hunched over or have that hump on their backs? That's what osteoporosis does. It is what ultimately destroys posture. It is a result of high-level loss of bone density, risking fracture and spinal degeneration. This happens usually to older people, mostly women. This condition can result in compression fractures wherein one or more vertebrae, usually on the lower thoracic or upper lumbar spine, compress or flatten out causing severe pain. As it heals, a *kyphotic or hump* posture develops.

It is assumed that taking calcium can slow it down but that's often not the solution. It's not really a lack of calcium that is the problem. It's caused by the acidic diet that we often have that leaches calcium out of the body along with decreased hormonal levels of estrogen. Taking medication such as estrogen hormone and *bisphosphonates* can help slow it down and even reverse it. However, more studies should be conducted to know if this is exactly true.

If you've turned on the TV lately, leafed through a magazine, or surfed the internet, you've likely seen an advertisement warning you about bone loss. The ad most likely recommends a certain medication to prevent it. It's true that many more people are suffering from osteoporosis today than in the past, but lots of women want to know if they really need to take Fosamax, Actonel, Boniva or some other prescription medication to strengthen their bones.

Some doctors say no to drugs. In almost all cases, taking a prescription medication is unnecessary. Even taking calcium will not prevent osteoporosis because it's not strictly a calcium problem. Anyway, many of us have enough calcium in our diets.

In 2004, the Surgeon General studied osteoporosis in the United States and wrote a report more than 330 pages long on the best ways to promote bone health and prevent osteoporosis and fracture. His advice, in essence, is to work with nature.

According to research, there is a prevalence of osteoporosis among underweight people, and overweight people are usually not at risk for this condition. In conclusion, bone density is improved by weight bearing exercises. So to prevent the occurrence of osteoporosis, go to a gym and lift weights especially if you're a woman of post-menopausal age.

Also an alkaline diet is essential as this promotes absorption of calcium and other minerals by the bone. A tablespoon of spirulina, wheatgrass or other grasses found in the health food store twice a day will help alkalize your body, as will eating mostly fruits and vegetables.

Piriformis Syndrome

It is also known as the "Fat Wallet Syndrome". This is the condition that is probably the most misdiagnosed as a disc herniation. The piriformis muscle goes across the buttocks. The sciatic nerve, which goes from the spine down the leg to the foot, exits through this muscle in 20 percent of the population. Spasm of this muscle, whether caused by injury or posture issues, can pinch and irritate the sciatic nerve. The symptoms are similar to a disc bulge—pain down the leg.

> *Quick Tip:*
>
> Don't wear your wallet in your back pocket. It will cause you to lean to one side when sitting and causes structural postural imbalances. However wearing a 1/8 or ¼ inch heel lift under one or the other side of the heel of your shoe can correct for leg length inequality or pelvic unleveling. See your chiropractor or physical therapist for this condition because the short leg could not really be short but rather the pelvis is rotated or high on one side making the leg appear shorter on one side when its not.

Jose M., a patient, underwent a disc surgery but still had these symptoms. I discovered that he had piriformis syndrome. I worked on relaxing his piriformis muscle through massage and stretching, and the symptoms disappeared.

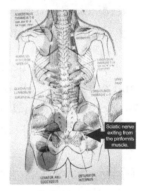

Sciatic nerve exiting from the piriformis muscle

Psoriatic Arthritis

This is an autoimmune disease that is best known for its skin lesions where the skin grows too fast and then sloughs off and causes lesions. People with this condition sometimes develop large bone spurs on the spine. However the joints remain intact and any pain from this is easily treated with chiropractic, physical therapy and exercises. Anti-inflammatory drugs can help reduce the initial pain.

Referral Pain

Although it happens rarely, back pain can come from non-back or spine related issues that can be serious such as:

1. Kidney infection or stones

2. Bladder infection

3. Bone cancer

4. Gall bladder stones

5. Pancreatitis

6. Cancer in any of the abdominal organs or prostate

These pains can be differentiated by different pain across the back that is not affected by little movements. However, sometimes they do mimic mechanical or extended back pain for weeks. It is very important to see your doctor to rule out these causes, should you feel any pain. Also if you feel other symptoms such as nausea, vomiting, malaise, fever or abdominal pain, see your doctor.

Rheumatoid Arthritis (RA)

This disease is totally different from osteoarthritis. This happens when the body has an autoimmune problem. What is an autoimmune problem? It is a problem wherein the cells of the body don't recognize its own kind. As a result, the cells attack and destroy the body's own cartilage in the joints. This disease doesn't exclusively affect the spine; it affects all the joints in the body, especially the joints of the hands, feet and the other joints of the extremities. Even worse is when the body's organs are affected like the kidneys. This causes great inflammation in the joints resulting in pain and instability. This can only be controlled by steroids, but other anti—inflammatory drugs such as Remicade are coming out and may prove to work much better.

Diet and food allergies can play a factor in this too. Eating foods that are devoid in gluten and foods that are anti-inflammatory help a lot with this. See Chapter 6 for more on diet.

> **Did You Know?**
> Remicade and other similar drugs are relatively new wonder drugs that are fairly natural and have very few side effects. You get one injection every one or two months. Sounds good doesn't it? Be aware it can cost $8,000 a shot! One of its side effects, however, is back pain. But that is rare. It's still an amazing drug for autoimmune diseases causing joint pain.

Sacroiliac Dysfunction

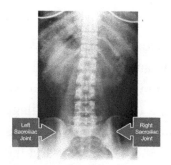

Picture of sacroiliac joint

This is when one has pain in the sacroiliac joint of the lower back; the pain can be in one or both sides of the lower back. Some folks call this the hips, but it is not. This dysfunction is due to a pelvis that's too far *posterior*. Bending forward, as you do at the bathroom sink, for example, will cause this. It usually manifests as deep pain that is made worse by flexion or bending forward. Arching backward to the side with the pain can bring relief. This condition is very responsive to physical rehab exercises, chiropractic manipulation and anti-inflammatory drugs.

Stenosis

This is a medical term that means a narrowing of a passage due to osteoarthritis. This is the result of too much arthritis and formation of bone spurs. In this condition, nerve impingements are almost always present. The passage where the nerve root exits (and in worst cases the spinal canal itself that holds the spinal cord) closes up. This is the

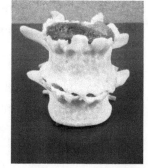

Stenosis—see the disc thinning and spurs which pinch the nerve coming out of the spine

worst type of back arthritis. Not only is it very hard to rehabilitate, it also needs to be managed with medications and surgery.

Subluxation

A subluxation is an incomplete dislocation or, more accuratley, joint dysfunction. It refers to a joint injury where a spinal joint becomes "stuck" and unable to move as freely as it should or becomes too mobile. This may occur with or without trauma.

A very well respected spine researcher, Dr Stuart McGill from The University of Waterloo in Canada, noticed in his research of an X-ray motion of a weight lifter that a single joint, upon lifting weights, moved too much compared to the other joints due to damage at that spot. There were also other subjects showing a single joint fixed in one spot as they lifted weights while all the other joints moved as they should. It's like driving a car where one wheel is misaligned and doesn't move freely, while the others do. Of course that tire will wear out faster and bulge or go bald as you drive. This is called joint dysfunction or *subluxation* and can eventually lead to many other back conditions including disc bulges and degeneration or arthritis. This subluxation/ dysfunction is more common than any other back condition and is typically corrected by a chiropractic adjustment.

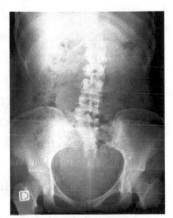
Misaligned spine

Sprain/Strain

A sprain/strain is where the ligaments that act like glue and hold the spine together and the muscles and tendons that attach to the spine are damaged and inflamed. Its healing period is often mistakenly assumed to be six weeks, but it's usually not. It may lead to joint dysfunction and to early arthritis, even though it appears that the pain is gone in six to twelve weeks. You'll see this as a result of car accidents, sports injuries, and lifting too much weight, especially when done incorrectly.

If the low back sprain or strain is serious, the doctor may recommend a day or two of rest, cold and/or heat therapy, and medications. Medications may include an anti-inflammatory to reduce swelling, a muscle relaxant to calm spasm, and a painkiller (narcotic) to alleviate intense but short-lived pain (acute pain). Most sprains and strains are pain free within a few weeks, but as said before the damage shows up later in a few years as arthritis.

Mild to moderate pain may be treated with non-steroidal anti-inflammatory drugs (NSAIDs). These work by relieving both swelling and pain. Many NSAIDs are available over-the-counter. Discuss the use of NSAIDs with your physician first.

The chiropractic and physical therapy approach to treating sprains and strains includes specific, gentle adjustments (also called spinal manipulations) or mobilizations to help restore spinal function. Stretches are also recommended to increase flexibility. If treatment is not performed arthritis can develop ten times faster, even if the pain disappears. I constantly see patients come in ten years after a car accident with big arthritic spurs in the neck or back because they never got this dysfunction completely fixed even though they were not in pain in the last ten years. I can estimate the date of the accident by the size of the spurs.

I had a patient Ronald S. who came in with severe neck pain that just came on that week. I took an X-ray and found giant spurs in his lower neck. I asked "Were you in a car accident 20 years ago?", and he said, "Oh yes I forgot. I got in a moderate fender bender 18 years ago. Why?" "I can tell by the size of the arthritic spurs," I said.

Trigger Point Pain

Trigger points are tender points in muscles, which are usually due to postural stress. However, they can also be from trauma caused by vehicular accidents or by lifting too much weight. When mismanaged, these muscle points can cause referred pain down the leg or across the gluteal area. They can mimic a pinched nerve, but are easy to fix with just very deep massage to pressure points along the back and gluteal area. Stretching the muscles in the back and gluteal area can also be of great help, along with applying heat for 20 minutes (no longer).

Summary:

There are many types of back pain from sprains to arthritis. You need to know what you have to be able to treat it correctly. ***Back problems can arise from mechanical injuries such as car accidents, by wear and tear or from autoimmune disorders such as Rheumatoid Arthritis****. Your medical doctor, chiropractor or physical therapist will be able to tell which one you have and how to treat it best. Most of the time, however,* ***back pain is caused by mechanical issues such as wear and tear, injury and postural issues****.*

Before you can find a way to deal with or eliminate your back pain, ***it must be identified****. Too often people self diagnose themselves incorrectly and end up making the problem worse with their efforts to "cure" themselves. Once you do find what your issue might be, you need to follow your doctor's guidelines for care or you will either worsen the original problem or create a whole new one.*

Your body must be structurally sound to work correctly. If there is an underlying problem with your foundation, you will have aches and pains that only get worse with time as the body compensates for the issue. ***Learn the causes and symptoms of the common back problems but do not try to diagnose initial or new symptoms on your own****.*

5

Look After Your Back and It Will Look After You

Possible Range of Treatments

There is no shortage of treatments for lower back issue. But most don't treat the underlying causes so they fail to have long-term relief. Here is a list of available treatments for back pain.

Typical Medical Treatment for Back Pain

Drugs or Medications

Drugs are usually the first answer! To accurately and most effectively treat your back pain, your doctor will need to make a diagnosis. Prior to doing anything else, he or she will have to determine what spinal condition is causing your back pain. With that information, he or she will be better able to prescribe medications to deal with your symptoms.

The medications should be part of a larger treatment plan that must include other treatment options such as chiropractic care, physical therapy, exercises and postural training. In other words, medication alone is not the ultimate solution to your back pain.

The severity and cause of your back pain determines the prescription for medications or injections. The ultimate goal should be to wean off medication.

Before we go into drugs for back pain, there is one misconception that I want to clarify. Because of TV advertisements, most people think that drugs are safe, effective and well understood. On the contrary, they're one of the most hazardous and poorly understood modes of treatment. Sometimes, they have adverse effects that are not fully established before they go out in the market.

One very good example of this is the COX-2 Inhibitors known as Celebrex, Vioxx and Bextra. They are non- steroidal anti-inflammatory drugs (NSAIDs) and at one point they were thought of as wonder drugs. They were supposed to be taken only for a month or less. However in cases where pain continued to be felt because of the fact that the real cause of the pain was not treated, doctors continued to prescribe them. Some people took the medication for years.

Years of intake of COX-2 Inhibitors took its toll and caused the deaths of a number of people due to heart disease and stroke, conditions that were later discovered to be closely associated with taking this drug.

Dr. Garret FitzGerald, a cardiologist and pharmacologist at the University of Pennsylvania, and his team of researchers have indicated that the COX-2 inhibitor painkillers may cause fatal heart disease.

The National Cancer Institute, which was conducting a long-term cancer study for Pfizer, also found that patients taking 400mg to 800mg of Celebrex daily had a 2.5 times greater risk of major heart problems than those who were taking placebos (look-alike pills with no active ingredients).

The Cleveland Clinic also conducted a study. This study appeared in the Journal of the American Medical Association. The study indicated that Celebrex (celecoxib) and Vioxx (rofecoxib) increased the annual rates of heart attack to more than 48,000 patients.

In 1994, Vioxx was taken off the market followed by Bextra. Celebrex on the other hand, is the only one of its kind that is still out in the market. It's still widely prescribed despite its adverse effects.

Chiropractic and physical therapy care are a thousand times safer and more effective than using medications to treat back pain. I wrote a study in the Journal of Manipulative Therapy (Vol 18, number 8 Oct 1995) to show this. To understand this, let's look at aspirin, the most common drug taken in the world. Did you know that aspirin has been used all the way back to around 400 B.C.? It's true! The father of modern medicine, Hippocrates, who lived sometime between 460 B.C. and 377 B.C., left records of pain treatments. And these historical records included the use of a powerful substance from the bark of the willow tree to treat fever, headache and various pains.

It wasn't until 1829 when scientists discovered that it was the compound called salicin from the willow plant that was in charge of the pain relief. In that same year, scientists were able to turn salicin into salicylic acid. The problem with salicylic acid, which limited its use, was the fact that it was too coarse for the stomach and the mouth to take. Then, in 1853, a German scientist named Gerhardt buffered it. Although it worked, it was excessively time consuming to prepare. He stopped preparing it, deeming it not worth the time

> **Did You Know?**
> During that same year (1897), Hoffmann synthesized heroin by accident.

In 1897, a German pharmacist named Felix Hoffmann who was working for a German pharmaceutical company, Bayer, started looking for a solution for his father's rheumatism. He recovered Gerhardt's work, and two years later in 1899, patented a "new" pain reliever under the name Aspirin.

But one of the truly remarkable things about all this is that scientists did not have a clue how aspirin worked until 1971. In that year, John Vane theorized how it worked and was awarded a Nobel Prize in 1982 for this work. His theory remains only a theory to this day.

Currently, 70 million pounds of aspirin are produced annually all over the world, making it the world's most widely used drug… and scientists *still* hypothesize about the exact mechanisms of aspirin. The point is, aspirin was given out without knowing how it works for more than a century because it got results.

Many drugs are given for back pain and what they do to the body are not well understood, and the dangers are not either.

Now drugs in general are safe, but my point is use them with caution. Pay attention to side effects, for you are the one who is taking the risk. Use them for short periods of time, and work on the real cause of the pain through diet, exercises, and corrective postural changes and also change or omit any of your activities that make it worse. That way you're not just treating the symptom by covering up the pain only.For covering up the pain only can lead to greater injury and degenerative changes. Pain is there for a reason, listen to it and act appropriately and responsibly.

> ### Did You Know?
> Although your doctor is an expert in medications, so is the pharmacist. Sometimes pharmacists will know the drugs better than anyone and it's free to ask them. So visit your local pharmacist for information and possible side effects if mixed with other prescriptions.

Your Doctor Might Prescribe

A: Over-the-Counter Medications for Back Pain

- *Acetaminophen*: Tylenol is an example of an acetaminophen, a type of medication that has proven to be a good pain reliever.

Your doctor may call this an analgesic, but most of us refer to acetaminophen medications as painkillers. They don't help reduce inflammation, though.

- *Over-the-counter NSAIDs* (non-steroidal anti-inflammatory drugs): These are best known as Advil, Motrin, Ibuprofen and Aleve. These you can take over the counter at 200-800 milligrams. But ask your medical doctor first if these are wise to take, and how much you should take. NSAIDS differ from acetaminophen because they help reduce swelling (they are anti-inflammatory) while relieving your pain. If an over-the-counter NSAID is an option for you, you have plenty to choose from.

According to some independent researchers, non-steroidal anti-inflammatory drugs, although generalized as not being harmful, are causing 20,000 deaths a year, so take great caution in taking them. They even double your chances of heart attacks.

There is also new evidence from the Cleveland Clinic study and The Lancet that showed taking anti-inflammatory medicine or cortisone shots or epidurals will slow down healing and those who did not take anti-inflammatory medicine have better long-term results and healing. That's because swelling causes the body to go into "insulin-like growth factor-1" and this speeds up muscle and other soft tissue healing.

Most athletes are aware of the RICE rule (rest, ice, compression and elevation) for dealing with minor strains and sprains. However, a study published in October, 2010 by the researchers at Cleveland Clinic has shown that swelling can play an important role in healing soft-tissue injuries. The study states that, "The result is a classic tradeoff between short-term and long-term benefits: reducing swelling with ice or anti-inflammatory drugs may ease your pain now, but slow down your ultimate return to full strength.[1]"

---

1   Hutchinson, Alex. *The Globe and Mail*. November 12, 2010. http://m.theglobeandmail. com/life/health/alex-hutchinson/take-a-pass-on-the-advil-swelling-may-help-you-heal/article1808598/?service=mobile

The study published in the *Journal of the Federation of American Societies for Experimental Biology* (FASEB Journal) essentially shows us the double-edged effects of anti-inflammatory drugs.

The study found that over-the-counter non-steroidal anti-inflammatories (NSAIDs) such as ibuprofen and ASA have been found to delay the eventual healing of tendon, muscle and ligament injuries.

What this means is that these medications bring initial relief for minor injuries, but there have been significantly worse outcomes a couple of months down the line.

B. Doctor Prescribed Medications

Muscle Relaxants: If you have chronic back pain caused by muscle spasms, you may need to take a muscle relaxant, which will help stop the spasms. These medications can make you drowsy, so they are not to be taken before driving. As mentioned earlier, muscle spasm is a protective mechanism. When there is damage or injury in the body, the muscles surrounding the damage go into spasms to splint the joints and prevent them from excessive movements that may cause more harm to the already injured tissues. Therefore, muscle relaxants will not have long-term affects and are quite often used way too much. Most of the time it's an inflammation problem, not a muscle problem. The muscles are doing their job by spasming and holding the back together so it does not move excessively.

Anti-depressants: As surprising as it may seem, anti-depressants can be effective for treating pain because they block pain messages on their way to the brain. They can also help increase your body's production of endorphins, which are the body's natural painkillers.

Opioids: In the most extreme cases, and only under careful supervision, your doctor may also prescribe an opioid, such as morphine or codeine.

Morphine-based drugs such as Oxycontin and Percocet work to reduce pain, but can be highly addictive. Tylenol is not addictive and may work better to reduce the pain, but is weaker than morphine-based drugs and does nothing for inflammation and spasms.

Be careful with painkillers because pain always has an underlying cause so you have to take care of the true cause of the pain and not just mask it with painkillers if you want permanent relief. In addition, without the pain, we will tend to move the injured part excessively, which will cause more damage.

As I was writing this section on drugs, I had a patient Gary D. who died from Oxycontin, a painkiller. He abused the drug and overdosed on it. The overdose caused over excretion of saliva, which cause him to drown. He was taking the drugs to kill his back pain from a surgery that had gone badly. What a tragedy!

> ### Quick Tip:
> Medication Warning—As with all medications, you must follow your doctor's advice precisely. Never mix over-the-counter and prescribed drugs or alcohol without consulting your doctor. Also, as your doctor decides what to prescribe, be sure to tell him or her if you're using any herbal supplements in addition to any other prescription medications you're taking.

Steroids: Actual steroids, such as a *Medrol* steroid pack for example, are good at reducing inflammation. Typically you take these for five to seven days in decreasing amounts every day. I have seen this work well for patients with severe back pain. But again, realize it may not have a good long-term outcome because swelling and pain cause the body to go into healing mode faster. I think medication, steroid or non-steroid, must be accompanied by rehab exercises and posture education for work, rest and play.

Summary of Medication: Drugs are usually the first line of defense against back pain and can help, but never really treat the cause. Quick solutions are what we're looking for, but back pain takes months and years to develop even though you may have just started to feel the back pain recently. Quick fixes are like changing a bald tire on a car without aligning the wheel that made it go bald in the first place, you will need to have it changed again soon.

Steroid Injections (ESI)

Epidural steroid injections have been used since 1952, and today are one of the most common treatment options for low back pain and leg pain. They target the epidural space, which is the space surrounding the membrane that covers the spine and nerve roots. Nerves travel through the epidural space and then branch out to other parts of your body, such as your legs. If a nerve root is compressed (pinched) in the epidural space, you can have pain that travels down your back and into your legs (commonly called sciatica, although the technical medical term is radiculopathy). The purpose of the injection is pain relief. Sometimes the injection alone is sufficient in providing pain relief, however it is best administered in combination with chiropractic or physical rehabilitation programs to provide long-term improvement.

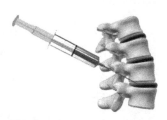

Epidural steroid injection

An epidural steroid injection sends steroids—which are very strong anti-inflammatory drugs—right to the nerve root that's inflamed. This is a pain management therapy, so it's best to have a well-trained pain management specialist do the injection. You'll probably need two or three injections. Generally, you shouldn't have more than that because of the potential side effects of the steroids.

How Does an Epidural Steroid Injection Work?

Prior to the injection, the area to be injected is anesthetized by a local anesthetic to numb it. Then the epidural steroid injection is performed. A steroid is injected directly around the dura, or the sac around the nerve roots that contains cerebrospinal fluid (the fluid around the brain, spinal cord and nerve roots).Injecting around the dural sac with steroids can markedly decrease inflammation associated with common conditions such as spinal stenosis, disc herniation or degenerative disc disease. It is thought that there is also a flushing effect from the injection that helps remove or "flush out" inflammatory proteins from around structures that may cause pain.

Epidural Steroid Injection Success Rates

An epidural steroid injection (ESI) is generally successful in relieving lower back pain for approximately half of the patients. The effects of the ESI tend to be temporary, ranging from a period of one week to one year, can be very beneficial in providing relief for patients during an episode of severe back pain and allows patients to progress in their rehabilitation. But the chances of epidurals by themselves eliminating a back problem or pain long term is five to ten percent.

But again, realize it may not have a good outcome for the long term because swelling and pain cause the body to go into healing mode faster. I believe that all drug-based treatments, including ESI, should be used with chiropractic care or physical therapy as well education about proper posture.

Other Injections

Depending upon your diagnosis, your doctor may suggest other types of spinal injections. For example, you can have a *sympathetic nerve block*, which targets the nerves that control some of your body's involuntary functions such as blood flow, temperature, sweating etc. The sympathetic nerves control things such as opening and closing blood vessels. A sympathetic nerve block involves an injection of drugs that numb the sympathetic nerves in the low back or neck. As a result the sympathetic nerves are "shut down" in the hopes of achieving pain relief.

You may also have a *facet joint injection.* Facet joints are the joints that connect our vertebrae. They make movement possible in the spine while providing stability as well. If they become inflamed, there will be pain. A facet joint injection will numb the joint and can reduce pain.

There is no definitive research that can tell us the ideal frequency of epidural steroid injections or other injections; however, a limit of three injections per year is generally considered reasonable. There is also no general consensus in the medical community as to whether or not a series of three injections always needs to be performed. If one or two injections resolve the patient's low back pain, some physicians prefer to save the one or two additional injections for any potential recurrences.

Epidural injections should ALWAYS be combined with chiropractic care, physical therapy, and posture training for they do not treat the cause, only the symptoms.

Medical doctors who understand back pain say taking NSAIDS and steroid anti-inflammatory drugs, which we discussed earlier, are better than taking painkillers and muscle relaxants or a combination of both. However, no matter what drug you take, you should always try to reverse the cause and not just eliminate the pain. This is where other forms of care such as proper posture training, physical therapy, chiropractic, exercise, massage and yoga can help.

> *Quick Tip:*
> Surgery is an invasive procedure, so always get two or three opinions before making your decision.

Surgery

Thank God for the surgeon I say. I know it's hard to believe I am saying that but when nothing else works this can be a lifesaver. However keep in mind 50% of the time after surgery the back problem comes back, not to mention many other complications like infection, chronic pain, and advanced scar tissue formation from the knife. These days, surgeons seem more understanding and more conservative than ever. This is crucial for surgery to work. I have seen patients have surgery because they waited too long for care. These days, surgeons do small incisions and work with lasers and do minimum actual surgery. Remember to have surgery is a last resort. A small piece of the herniated disc may be removed, or spurs shaved off. Sometime more complex surgery such as a spinal fusion is necessary, but this should not be the norm. These are done by neurosurgeons and orthopedists. I do not like hardware used where metal screws and braces are being left in a patient. This only should happen with very unstable backs. Remember surgery always needs to be followed by physical therapy, chiropractic and posture training program to strengthen and prevent more back issues.

You may be fearful of back surgery, but in fact, only one to two percent of people need surgery to treat back problems. Your pain may be severe, but most sprains and strains do not require surgery. Surgery is reserved for the most severe cases of back pain (spinal cord impingement, structural deformity, severe cases of spinal stenosis).

In most case surgery should be considered only after you've tried several months of non-surgical treatment. Many surgical procedures can be performed using minimally invasive techniques, which means less "cutting" or entering the body. These techniques result in smaller incisions, shorter hospital stays, less pain after surgery, and a faster recovery.

Some Typical Spinal Surgeries Include:

Facetectomy: A procedure that removes a part of the facet (a bony structure in the spinal canal) to increase the space.

Foraminotomy: A procedure that removes the foramina (the area where the nerve roots exit the spinal canal) to increase the size of the nerve pathway. This surgery can be done alone or with a laminotomy.

Laminoplasty: A procedure that reaches the cervical spine (neck) from the back of the neck, which is then reconstructed to make more room for the spinal canal.

Laminotomy: A procedure that removes only a small portion of the lamina (a part of the vertebra) to relieve pressure on the nerve roots.

Micro-discectomy: A procedure that removes a disc through a very small incision using a microscope.

Spinal Laminectomy: A procedure for treating spinal stenosis by relieving pressure on the spinal cord. A part of the lamina (a part of the vertebra) is removed or trimmed to widen the spinal canal and create more space for the spinal nerves.

I had a patient Aaron R who wanted back surgery for a minor disc bulge because he wanted it fixed fast. It helped right away, but six months later he was back in to see me because scar tissue had developed from the original injury and possibly the surgery itself. In the end, he got better with proper conservative care and rehab, and his back stayed healthy for years.

Don't wait too long for more invasive care such as surgery, if it's warranted. I had a patient Eve W. who did not want surgery and now has permanent foot drop. Every time she takes a step her foot slaps on the ground.

Typical Non Medical or Alternative Treatment for Acute Low Back Pain

Did You Know?
In 1997, Americans spent $27 billion on alternative therapies. Nearly a third of the country's population, 83 million people, partook of alternative therapies to improve their health.

Typical non medical or alternative treatment for acute low back pain are the problems that western medicine has to solve urgently today. These changes remind us that human beings are still part of nature, and need holistic solutions rather than just chemical fixes. Thus, eastern medicine, which has proven itself for more than two thousand years, once again stands out. The whole world turns to eastern approaches to take us away from pain and keep us young by natural approaches. It is called alternative medicine—also folk therapy, in Chinese.

A century ago, alternative medicine was not yet accepted by science yet. Until the mid-1990s, it was still not granted the same respect as mainstream medicine. Senator Tom Harkin noted that we do not pay enough attention to alternative medicine and that we should change our beliefs and behaviors to prevent diseases and take care of our own health. Alternative medicine remains unshakable and gains ground as time goes by because it works.

> **Did You Know?**
>
> 63% of Our Maladies Can Be Cured by the Body's Natural Defense System
>
> *Source: Statistics from WHO*

Listed below are effective treatments for back pain. They relieve pain by fixing its real causes.

Chiropractic

Chiropractic is a branch of alternative medicine that is based on the concept that all of the body's functions are correlated to the nervous system. Chiropractic involves manipulations and/or adjustments of body structures, such as the spinal column, so that pressure on nerves coming from the spinal cord due to displacement (subluxation) of a vertebral body may be relieved.

A chiropractor is a highly specialized rehabilitation specialist known best for joint manipulation. This is shown by many American workers compensation studies and by British, Canadian and Australian researchers as well as those in many other countries to be twice as effective for treating back pain. According to the Governments of USA, England, Germany, Canada and many US state Worker Compensation studies, chiropractic treatment for back pain is better than medicine and physical therapy and gets people to return to work twice as fast. However, without the physical therapy rehabilitation exercises, the problem or pain can come back. What is not well known is that most chiropractors are trained in rehabilitative exercises such as posture training, massage and trigger point therapy, which when combined with back manipulation are very powerful forms of back care. They're even up to 1,000 times safer than medications and surgery.

Joint manipulation is a powerful treatment because very often-back pain comes from joint dysfunctions in the lower back where the joints are not moving properly. When the joints are not moving properly, they can swell, cause pain, degenerate and build up scar tissue, then eventually calcium deposits or spurs will be formed. When this all combines, it will lead to arthritis. See your joints if injured or over time are like door hinges and eventually they rust. Eventually the door is hard to open and close and squeek and if left in the rain it can eventually get stuck and immovable.

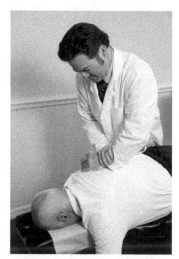

Chiropractic treatment

Manipulation is where the joint is lightly moved beyond normal physiological stretch and it produces an audible pop, like cracking your knuckles. It feels good, and your hands move more easily afterwards. The same is true with the back. However, the back has an additional benefit of creating a feedback loop with a spinal recurring nerve that relaxes the muscles in the spine. It then creates mobility in a fixated stuck joint, like adding oil to a rusty hinge.

So how do you fix a rusty door hinge? You add oil and force it open and closed many times to creat mobility and grind away the rust. This is the same concept to Chiropractic manipulation. That popping noise is nitrogen gas and fluid going into the joint space-acting like oil and creats movement to a stuck joint. It can give instant relief as I have seen thousands of times. *"Ahh, that feels much better after that pop"* my patients say all the time. Manipulation can stop and reverse this stuck or arthritic joint depending on the severity, but it needs to be done repetitively two or three times a week for six to twelve weeks so that normal joint mobility returns with normal tissue recovery. It allows normal tissue and fluid to grow back from the scar tissues that caused the joint to get stuck in the first place.

Chiropractors take five years postgraduate doctorate training that's similar to medical school but puts more emphasis on joint mechanics and rehabilitation and less on medicine and surgery. They all need a license to practice in every state and all western countries, like a medical doctor and dentist. When looking for a chiropractor, ask if they do osseous manipulation, rehabilitative exercises and posture training. This is the best trio combo I know to fix a back—unless it's too far gone and a surgeon is needed.

Did You Know?

In 1994 the UK and the US almost simultaneously published official guidelines for the treatment of acute low back pain. Both documents stipulated the utilization of spinal manipulation, a primary form of chiropractic treatment, as a first choice in the treatment for acute low back pain. Now, for the first time, a non-chiropractic group had recommended chiropractic based on research data that overwhelmingly supported spinal manipulation as an effective, safe and less expensive form of care compared to all the other treatment approaches that the health care consumer can choose. According to the published guidelines, ALL patients with acute AND chronic low back pain should see chiropractors FIRST.

Physical Therapy

This is a practice similar to chiropractic, but it does not use manipulation. Instead it makes use of joint mobilization and rehabilitative exercises. Mobilization is gentle stretching without the pop. Physical therapists emphasize good postural mechanics and exercises to strengthen key muscles and stretch tight muscles. They also do modalities such as muscle stimulation, heat to relax muscles, ultrasound and laser to break up scar tissue, and traction to stretch out the back. Many chiropractors use these modalities as well. Modalities such as these can help reduce acute pain. Long-term relief will not be achieved without rehabilitative exercises and posture training. Many times however, posture training is not done accurately and patients are taught with methods reflecting how most of us are in western society. But we need to learn the posture the underdeveloped societies such as a typical Haitian or African tribal person whose posture has been unchanged for centuries. This will be discussed later in Chapter 7.

Physical therapy training takes three years, and a fourth year can be added for the new doctorate degree.

Heat and Cold Therapy

During the first 24 to 48 hours after an injury, cold therapy helps to reduce swelling, muscle spasm and pain by reducing blood flow to the injured area. Never apply cold or ice directly to skin. Instead wrap the ice pack or cold product in a towel and apply for no longer than 10 minutes.

Usually, after the first 48 hours, heat therapy is used to warm sore tissues. Never apply heat directly to skin; instead, wrap the heat source in a thick towel. Heat increases blood flow, warming and relaxing soft tissues. Heat therapy is often used in physical therapy to increase flexibility prior to gentle stretching and exercise. Never use heat for more than 20 minutes or ice for more than 10 minutes or it will cause more inflammation. When combined with stretching, the benefits of heat therapy are greater than heat alone.

Modalities

There are five kinds of physical therapies and chiropractic modalities commonly used on the low back to help reduce spasm, inflammation and pain. These do not work well on their own and need to be used with exercises, manual therapy or spinal manipulation and posture training.

There are five main kinds:

- Electrical Stimulation
- Ultrasound
- Mechanical Traction
- Decompression Therapy
- Cold Laser

Electrical Stimulation

Electrical stimulation uses an electrical current to cause a single muscle or a group of muscles to contract. By placing electrodes on the skin in various locations, the physical therapist can recruit the appropriate muscle fibers.

Contracting the muscle via electrical stimulation helps strengthen the affected muscle. The physical therapist can change the current setting to allow for a forceful or gentle muscle contraction. Along with increasing muscle strength, the contraction of the muscle also promotes blood supply to the area, which assists in healing.

> ***Quick Tip:***
>
> Do Not Use Electrical Stimulation, Traction or Ultrasound if You:
>
> - Have arrhythmia (You will need to be evaluated by Physician before using the unit.)
> - Have a pace maker
> - Have heart disease
> - Are pregnant
> - Have cancer

Five Main Kinds of Electrical Stimulation

1. Interferential
2. High Volt Galvanic
3. Low Volt Galvanic
4. Microcurrent
5. TENS

Interferential Therapy

A form of electro therapy, Interferential therapy is used in the treatment of muscle pain and injuries. This type of treatment uses mid-frequency electrical currents on the muscle, which helps heal injuries and relieve pain.

Essentially, how interferential therapy works is that it creates a current that has a massaging affect on the muscle; this in turn, helps to stimulate the release of endorphins, which is a natural pain reliever made by the body. This helps to relieve pain and also helps with healing injury to the soft tissue.

While interferential therapy is extremely effective in relieving pain of strained muscles, it is not recommended if there are any open wounds or injuries.

Uses:

- To treat and relieve and manage chronic pain
- As adjunctive treatment in the management of post surgical and post traumatic acute pain

High Volt Galvanic

Theoretically, high voltage galvanic uses direct current to create an electrical field over the treated area that changes blood flow. The positive pad behaves like ice, causing reduced circulation to the area under the pad and reduction in swelling. The negative pad behaves like heat, causing increased circulation, reportedly speeding healing. A high voltage device produces a spontaneous breakdown in skin resistance and currents pass through the skin with negligible thermal and electrochemical effects. By decreasing the pulse duration and increasing the voltage, the developers noted that deep tissues could be stimulated without producing tissue damage.

Used for:

- Pain relief (acute and chronic pain)
- Increase blood circulation, promote metabolism
- Muscle rehabilitation
- Help heal injury
- Edema reduction.
- Reduce inflammation

Low Voltage Galvanic

Direct current is utilized in low ampere ranges for the unique electro-chemical effects its unidirectional current provides.

Used for:

- Facilitating repair of injured or damaged tissue
- Reducing inflammation and pain
- Stimulating muscles

Microcurrent

Microcurrent is used for the relief of pain, because of its close proximity to our own body's current, and is thought to work on a more cellular level.

Microcurrent is measured in Micro Amps, millionths of an ampere.

It is theorized that healthy tissue is the result of direct flow of electrical current throughout the body. Electrical balance is disrupted when the body is injured at a particular site, causing the electrical current to change course. The use of microcurrent over the injured site is thought to realign this flow, thus aiding in tissue repair.

It has been found that ATP (Adenosine Triphosphate) in the cell helps promote protein synthesis and healing. The lack of ATP, due to trauma of the tissue, results in the decreased production of sodium and an increase in metabolic waste, which is perceived as pain. The use of microcurrent at an injured area helps realign the body's electrical current and increase the production of ATP, resulting in increased healing and recovery, as well as blocking the pain that is perceived. So in essence, the basis of electrotherapy is a direct transfer of electricity into the body to excite or steady the nerves.

Joanie Benoit, who set a record for the women's marathon in the 1984 Olympics, has used microcurrent to promote post-operative healing and relieve pain. Also, Joe Montana, the NFL football quaterback player, used microcurrent to help his back recover from surgery and went back to win more championships.

Used For:

- Chronic/ acute pain sufferer
- Promote blood circulation, relieve pain.
- Sports injury (soft tissue injuries, swelling and fractures)
- Firming and toning muscle
- Reduce signs of aging, for examples, wrinkles, scars, fine lines
- Wound healing

TENS

A TENS unit is a pocket size, portable, battery-operated device that sends electrical impulses to certain parts of the body to block pain signals. The origins of TENS (Transcutaneous Electrical Nerve Stimulator/ Stimulation) goes back to the doctors of the ancient Rome. They used electric eels to treat people who suffered from headaches and arthritis. Now in the high tech age, we have the TENS units. It is used to stimulate the nerve, muscle and cells via surface skin with a low electrical current to make the brain produce endorphins (natural pain killers) and then to reach the goal of relieving syndromes and stopping pain.

The electrical currents produced are mild and do not go as deep as in other stimulation therapies used in physical therapy and chiropractic offices, but they can prevent pain messages from being transmitted to the brain and may raise the level of endorphins.

TENS units should only be used under the direction of a doctor, chiropractor or physical therapist. Electrodes are attached to the surface of the skin over or near the area where you are experiencing pain.

It is important that you learn how to:

- Correctly put on the electrodes (proper placement is important)
- Operate the unit
- Change the batteries

- Vary the controls and settings (both the frequency and voltage)
- Set the proper duration and intensity of the stimulation (which depends on the location and type of pain)

The units can be purchased online for home use. The cost of a TENS unit can range from about $100 to several hundred dollars. TENS units can be purchased or rented. A prescription usually is necessary for insurance reimbursement of a TENS unit.

Research shows that a TENS unit works as well as a placebo, which means about ten percent of people with back pain will be helped by this, although it never fixes the back problem.

Used to: control pain

Ultrasound

Think of what the name implies; it is a kind of sound. Sound waves are like ripples with different sizes and densities. Different waves bring us sounds high and low. A human's hearing range is from 20 to 18000Hz (vibrations per second). The higher the Hz is, the higher the tone we hear. Like the strings of a violin, the thinnest one always produces the higher sound. Ultrasound is a sound that human beings cannot hear. In engineering, a rate over 20000Hz is called ultrasound.

To a human's hearing, ultrasound might mean nothing, while to many animals, it is heard clearly. If ultrasound means nothing to our hearing, what can we do with it? We can take the advantage of its density and speed on more subtle functions. First of all, we have to know what ultrasound can do.

These sound waves are transmitted to the surrounding tissue and vasculature. They penetrate the muscles to cause deep tissue/muscle warming. This promotes tissue relaxation and therefore is useful in treating muscle tightness and spasms. The warming effect of the sound waves also causes vessel vasodilatation and increases circulation to the area that assists in healing. Physical therapists and chiropractors can also adjust the frequency on the machine to use waves that will decrease inflammation.

In most cases, ultrasound does not work well with back pain, but is better with extremity problems such as tennis elbow.

Mechanical Traction

Traction is a modality sometimes given by physical therapists and chiropractors. The purpose of traction is to apply a force that draws two adjacent bones apart from each other in order to increase their shared joint space. Traction also stretches the soft tissue that surrounds the joint. Traction may be given manually, by means of a device or via positioning.

In the spine, the elongation provided by traction allows facet joints to slide, increases circulation and relieves pressure on the spinal cord, its blood vessels and nerve roots. The improved circulation has an added, indirect benefit of decreasing toxins in damaged tissues brought about by inflammation. The movement at the joints may also help decrease tension, which is another source of pain.

Traction may be given continuously for up to 10 minutes at a time or intermittently for up to 15 minutes. This experience is meant to provide relaxation to the patient, rather than more tension.

Although many people can attest to the fact that traction on the spine feels good, a 2005 review of medical literature by the Cochrane Back Group found that, by itself, traction really isn't effective for lower back pain. After looking at 25 high-quality studies, which investigated a total of more than 1,000 traction patients, researchers concluded that if you are using traction as the only treatment, there's really no difference in results between it and a placebo. For certain types of neck problems, though, the use of traction is alive and well in clinical settings, as a complement to other treatment measures.

I find mechanical traction works best for people with low back arthritis. It can be used for disc herniation, but it can aggravate the problem, thus I don't recommend lumbar traction for disc herniation unless all else fails and surgery is the only next option left. However there is a form of traction known as decompression therapy, which is relatively new. We will discuss this next.

Decompression Therapy

This is a relatively new form of care for low back pain. It is primarily done by chiropractors, but physical therapists and MDs can do it as well. It is a computerized form of traction that angles the traction with a complex harness and traction table to decompress only the section of the back that needs attention such as L5 - S1 disc herniation. The procedure may not be covered by health insurance and it is considered costly for 20-25 treatments. It is typically followed by some form of physical therapy such as muscle stimulation and ice.

Reports have been published stating that decompression therapy is 90% effective, but these are not verified with research. In my opinion, it works best with people with arthritis or chronic disc herniation, but is not as effective as chiropractic or physical therapy. However, if no other forms of care are helping, adding this may help and is perhaps be worth a try.

My patient Jim B., who was 68 years old, had moderate pain in his back, down both of his legs to his feet. An MRI showed all his lumbar vertebrae were degenerated so much that the spine looked deformed. They wanted to do surgery, but it would have been extensive and would leave him with rods and steel in his back. Instead, we tried decompression therapy on him. After six weeks, he was 80% better, and after 12 weeks, he was out

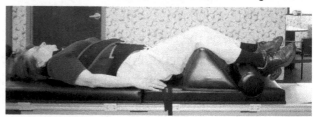

Decompression table –similar to traction but more powerful and isolates one area and decompresses that area only

of pain and had mild stiffness only. He could again enjoy walking in the park, and gardening.

Inversion Therapy

Discs separate vertebrae, allow movement and provide shock absorption. Dangerous exercises or constant pounding from running can cause the discs to be compressed. The centre of the disc contains a jelly type liquid which can protrude out and put pressure on the nerves. Inverted, your body weight applies mild traction to the spine which becomes slightly longer. This increases the space between the vertebrae and reduces the pressure on the discs. Every nerve in the body leaves the spine through the spaces between the vertebrae. Increasing the space between the vertebrae reduces the pressure on the nerve roots and discs, which means less back pain.

By hanging upside on an inversion table this antigravity action is created for fluids around the spinal discs forcing waste out and drawing in fluid around the discs. Inversion helps to relax muscles which increases blood flow through the muscles which in turn maintains the muscles in better condition and less likely to cause painful spasms. It has been found helpful for home therapy but there may be an increase of a stroke from hanging upside down so if you are prone to cardiovascular disease or high blood pressure I would not advise.

Cold Laser

Since its U.S. Food and Drug Administration (FDA) approval in 2002, cold laser treatment for pain relief has been popular for sufferers of chronic back pain. Cold lasers are used to trigger the body's natural healing response by penetrating the surface skin tissue to target the affected under-layers with low-energy infrared or near-infrared light. The energy stimulates the cells, "kick starting" the cell processes so that new, healthy cells are regenerated to replace the abnormal cells. The low-energy cell stimulation reduces pain and swelling and triggers the musculoskeletal abnormalities that cause the symptoms of pain and swelling to heal on their own. This occurs not only during treatment, but also between and after treatments. There are no known side effects.

Cold laser treatment is completely painless, and patients can generally continue on with their daily activities, since there is no downtime. The lasers used don't damage, cut or burn the skin.

Laser therapy is regarded within the medical profession and by the FDA as a safe and effective treatment for back pain. However, multiple sessions are needed for optimal performance, and Spine-Health.com reports that eight to 30 sessions may be required.

Exercises

Well this is one of my favorite ways to reduce, eliminate and prevent back pain because it deals with all the causes of back pain. Why? Because MOST back pain is caused by muscular and structural imbalance and that can be corrected with the right specific exercises.

There are Three Types of Exercises

Proprioceptive Exercises—Proprioception is our perception or awareness of where exactly our body and limbs are in space.

> **Did You Know?**
> Proprioception tests such as putting one foot in front of the other in a line while keeping balanced have been used by the police to determine whether drivers are drunk.

Proprioceptive exercises are about balance and communication between the brain and the rest of the body. Their purpose is to ensure that the back sends impulses to the brain and vice versa to help the smaller muscles guide proper posture and function. For example, the extensor or multifidi muscles are the deep muscles that run up and down your spine that hold up the integrity of your spine so it doesn't collapse forward. To accomplish this they have receptors or sensors in the fibers of each of the hundreds of tiny multifidi muscles that tell them how tight they should be. Too tight, and your spine overly extends too loose and the spine collapses. So the muscles are always firing, but to the perfect amount of tightness. These sensors are always registering the movement of the body and relaying messages to the brain and the muscles to the spine. In fact all muscles in the body have these sensors. This is known as the "stretch reflex" and it all happens at an unconscious level. It gives the muscle its "tone". This prevents the body from falling down and keeps the body erect. This activity of postural muscles serves as the background against which all-specific actions like walking, running, throwing a ball, take place.

Sometimes these sensors don't communicate properly with the brain and muscles and give false readings or are over or under stimulated by bad posture, caffeine or drugs. To correct for this we need balance exercises which make these muscles fire rapidly and makes the sensors work overtime and get "reset".

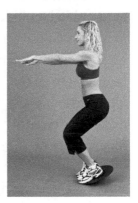

Balance exercising on a wobble board

For balance or proprioception exercises, we use a wobble board. If you step on a wobble board, you will feel the small multifidi muscles that run up and down both sides of the whole spine fire up rapidly from right to left and back again. We also use an exercise ball or just stand on one leg for 30 seconds eyes open then eyes closed Doing this on one leg at home for 1-3 minutes provides a more advanced proprioceptive exercise.

Stretching Exercises of Key Muscles—These are important because muscle tightness is a major cause of back pain. For example, tightness of the hamstring muscles shifts the pelvic posture, which causes back pain (See Chapter 2 for more details). In addition, other nerve impingements, such as piriformis syndrome are caused by muscle tightness and muscle spasms. (This is discussed in detail in Chapter 4). Therefore stretching exercises are imperative to treat back pain.

Mary S. was a patient of mine who had a failed disc surgery for her sciatica. The surgery didn't work because it wasn't the disc bulge that caused the sciatica, but piriformis syndrome, which pinched the nerve. We just stretched the piriformis muscle, and the sciatica went away. Stretching is the key to bringing back flexibility, and for back pain, the key muscles to be stretched are the hamstrings, the piriformis, the gluteals or buttock muscles, and the psoas or the hip muscles. Tight hamstrings and psoas muscles cause pressure to increase on the lower back resulting in disc herniation.

Strengthening Exercises of Weak Key Muscles are crucial to reduce and prevent back pain. Eighty percent of people with back pain have weak or atrophied multifidi muscles on one side of the lower back. These are the muscles that run up and down both sides of your spine. You can feel these muscles when you place your fingers on the bumps of your spine and then move them about an inch to the right or to the left. These muscles control the fine movements of the spine, and when they are weak on one side, spinal joint dysfunction will occur, which can lead to

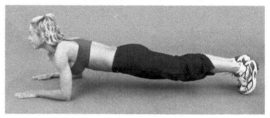

Plank exercises to help stabilize

disc herniation, arthritis and many other back conditions.

Most people with back problems have weak multifidi muscles and weak core muscles, which are the abdominals and muscles around the pelvis. To relieve their back pain, their core muscles need to be strengthened.

My expertise is exercise focused on proprioception, stretching and strengthening key muscles. I developed the "Dabbs Accelerated Back Care System" video on DVD. It has all the tips and the proven system you need so you can rehabilitate your back every day or every other day for 15-20 minutes with me in the leisure of your own home, and in six weeks or sooner, you will feel better.

Visit me at www.DrDabbs.com and get free tips. See the Dabbs Accelerated Back Care System tab or go to www.DrDabbs.com/Product to purchase the entire system, which includes all the equipment, such as

the exercise ball, wobble board, foam roller, elastic band, and the five-DVD system itself, which has developed over the last 23 years of practice and research. Medical doctors, chiropractors, physical therapists and physical trainers have tested this system over the years, and they can guarantee you that it works!

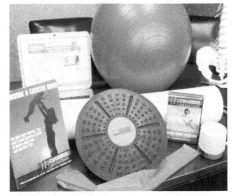

Dabbs accelerated back care system

Massage

Massage comes in various forms from light Swedish to deep pressure such as Rolfing and trigger point therapy. I happen to think trigger point therapy, Rolfing or deep tissue massage does more to break up scar tissues or knots. However for a sensitive person, Swedish is the next best thing. Massage, done three to five times on an area with pain and tension, can break up muscle and tendon knots and can create better muscle function, strength and flexibility. Sometimes the knots, also called trigger points or scar tissue, are the cause of pain and they can refer pain down the leg similar to the way a pinched nerve does. So, I always like to treat back pain with massage to relieve muscle tensions and pain.

The only caution in doing massage is if the patient has difficulty lying on his or her stomach for a period of time. When this is the case, make sure the massage is done while the patient is on his side or have a big pillow under the patient's pelvis to put his back in flexion to ease tension.

Home treatment with the use of a foam roller made of a semi firm foam is an option, which is a three feet long and six inches in diameter. You lie on it on your sore spots and roll back and forth to knead the sore spots out. It can be very powerful to remove trigger points or knots, especially in the buttocks, hip and back muscles. The more weight you put on the area, the more it kneads it, but do it at a comfortable weight and go slowly on the pressure. Do it daily for one or two weeks until your back feels better. You can buy a foam roller on my website www.DrDabbs.com/Product.

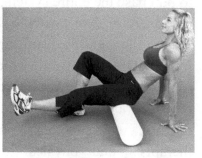

I had a patient Jennifer M. who had an annoying pain in her back muscles and I applied pressure with my thumb on a trigger point and massaged it for five minutes, after which she said felt better. I then told her to use the foam roller daily. She had more immediate relief that

Foam roller use for self massage—roll back and forth applying as much weight over the sore or tight muscle

continued until the trigger point knot in her buttocks was gone within a week. She was then pain free.

Yoga

Yoga was developed thousands of years ago in India as a gentle way to gain flexibility and strength. It utilizes proper posture mechanics and breathing techniques. It can be helpful for back pain, but it can also make it worse if you are not trained properly. Before engaging in yoga exercises, let your instructor know about your back problem and ask your doctor or chiropractor if it would be good for you, then start slowly and easily. Ask your friends and colleagues for recommendations for good yoga instructors in your area. There is no state licensing for yoga instructors, so word of mouth is a good way to find a competent instructor. Yoga will not have the effect you're looking for if you don't change and improve your daily posture.

I knew the owner of the largest yoga center in Maryland, and one day he came in as a patient with low back pain. Now this guy could wind his legs around his head even though he was 58 years old. We X-rayed him and saw giant spurs on every vertebra in his low back, yet he was extremely flexible. We treated him for a week and he was well. A normal person would have taken weeks or months to heal, but because he was a yoga instructor, his yoga helped keep his spine flexible, which is good for the back.

Pilates

Pilates is like yoga and weight lifting rolled into one. It is a combination of Eastern and Western exercises developed a century ago by Joseph Pilates. Pilates uses specific movement and equipment, and it is done at gyms or Pilates centers. It emphasizes proper posture, breathing, injury prevention, proper stretching and strengthening. The strengthening is for elongation of muscles, not bulk. It uses floor mats and a low level piece of equipment called a transformer, which is like a rowing machine with pulleys and ropes. Your abdominals or core muscles are the key to the workout along with balance, breathing and relaxation.

Hypnosis

Hypnosis is an art as well as a science. It was developed 200 years ago by Franz Anton Mesmer and is still in use for many medical and non-medical conditions. Back pain is not commonly treated with hypnosis, but that doesn't mean it won't help. It emphasizes relaxation and proper breathing with verbal or visual suggestions given by the hypnotist. Just the relaxation and breathing can help. The suggestions such as "your back pain is easing" may or may not work on everyone as some people just can't be hypnotized, but it may be worth a try if everything else is failing. Find a hypnotist who's a licensed psychologist, psychiatrist or therapist who has been well trained in hypnotherapy.

Biofeedback

With Biofeedback, the patient is hooked up to a computer that monitors his heart rate, muscle tension, skin temperature, galvanic skin response and brain waves. The patient will see visually on the monitor when the tension in his back is relieved by relaxation so he can train his mind to learn how to do this on his own without the use of the electrodes hooking him up to a computer. It was used more in the 1980s; however it seems to have limited success. If not much is working for your back pain and you tried exercises, medications, proper posture and other professionals such as chiropractors, physical therapists and massage therapists, acupuncture but nothing seems to work, then you can try biofeedback. I suggest five to fifteen sessions. Beware of practitioners who prescribe too many treatments.

Acupuncture

Acupuncture is an ancient Eastern medical treatment for many ailments.

I believe that there are four components to health: chemical, which involves nutrition and medicine; mechanical, which involves exercise, chiropractic alignment and posture; mental, which involves the mind; and electrical or energy, which includes acupuncture. All these components affect one another.

Acupuncture is based on the concept that the flow of energy follows specific lines along the body like wires in a building. These lines are called meridians, of which there are 14, and their function is not well understood but have been measured in studies.

The matter traveling on the meridians is the body energy called *chi*. These rivers of energy called chi surface at specific places in the skin. If there is a block, or the flow of energy is too great in one of these meridians, it can cause problems in the area of the body it specifically targets. It is the fountain of the life composed of ying and yang. **Yin and yang** in Chinese philosophy are opposite forces that form a whole. Everything contains both yin and yang in a balance that is always changing, such as hot and cold, day and night, and health and disease. In traditional Chinese medicine, disease is diagnosed and treated based on the balance of yin and yang. When chi flows through these meridian paths, it can change with the body motion and outside stimulation.

Placing needles or heated herbs known as *moxa* over these acupuncture points can restore the proper energy flow. Western medicine thinks these points release endorphins in the brain and this reduces pain.

I have had some patients get relief from this, but it's hit or miss. And if back pain is mechanical, which most is, then it stands to reason to fix that first through proper posture, exercises and the use of good mechanics.

Acupuncturists are usually licensed in the United States and other western countries and if you want to try, do it for six to twelve sessions. If you see no results, then try something else.

Meditation

There are 60,000 thoughts per minute going on in the brain. Stress causes muscles to tighten and restrict blood vessels. Meditation is where one lies or sits in a neutral spine posture and becomes very relaxed. One can lead oneself to a heightened spiritual realization called Samadhi, but even without this, it will let one's mind become relaxed and focused. It has been shown to lower blood pressure, reduce muscle tension, slow heart rate, slow brain wave activities, improve oxygen consumption, improve immune system function and reduce pain. It's free, so why not try it? Get a book or join a class and learn the best way to do this. It is worth a try to relieve your lower back pain.

Tai Chi

Tai Chi is an exercise involving slow controlled movements of the body, arms, legs, hands and feet with controlled breathing while coordinating with the mind. Its goal is to achieve calm and peace. This is also similar to Qi Qong and Aikido. This is an Eastern exercise where one does slow methodical movements while standing. It is similar to martial arts. This is great for balance and posture but must be done with an instructor who is well trained in traditional techniques and who himself has a good posture. It is a good exercise for all, most especially the elderly since it requires little strength and agility and can be performed as much as one wants. This exercise is worth trying for those who want to ease their back problem.

Home Care

Exercises in the form of stretching and strengthening, as well as heat or ice therapy can work in the comfort of your own home.

When you can't move due to acute pain, lie on the floor facing up, and put your legs on a chair and rest there for 30 minutes. This is called the *recovery position* and it really relaxes the back.

For a great home rehabilitation program, visit me at www.DrDabbs. com/product where you can get the "Dabbs Accelerated Back Care System". This is a system I developed from 22 years of experience and put together for you for a home based self treatment of your back pain. It is a great six-week program that puts all exercises together for you as a step-by-step guide. You can do it with me daily for six weeks in the comfort of your own home. I will take you through a simple exercise program at three different levels (beginners, intermediate and advanced). The exercises included there are focused on the key muscles and joints to improve flexibility, strength and balance so you can have a pain free and strong back.

Ice and heat are good home remedies for back pain. "So when do I use ice or heat?" I get asked this all the time. Well, if the back pain or any joint or muscle pain just occurred, especially from an injury; use ice for ten minutes right on the sore spot. Ice prevents swelling and numbs the pain. Use a paper towel that is not too thin or too thick between the ice and the skin to prevent skin burn. Do not apply ice for longer than ten minutes or the skin can blister. Ice will feel cold and painful for two minutes, after that you will go numb. So, just bear with ice for the first four minutes, and it will feel good after that.

After 24 hours, you can start using a combo of ice for ten minutes, followed by heat for 20 minutes, to be repeated every hour. This contracts and expands the tissue, forcing out the swelling.

If the injury is more than 48 hours old, use heat for 20 minutes and don't go any longer as it can cause blisters and more swelling.

Twenty minutes of heat will remove swelling, relax the muscles and help relieve the pain. Never sleep on a heating pad or it will swell the area like a balloon. You can use heat and ice every hour if you want throughout the day.

Diet

Diet plays an important part in decreasing inflammation, speeding healing and preventing disease. If medicine was truly a healing profession, it would concentrate first on diet and exercises which would save lives and increase the quality of life. Imagine if you went to your MD and he said for all conditions "well let's get you on a healthy diet and an exercise program and I will monitor it and I won't get paid until you do this and see results". Well they do this in socialized Europe and Canada where Doctors get paid more when they get patients to stop smoking, eat healthily and exercise and lose weight. More and more MDs now are doing this, but it's still rare. See Chapter 6 for details on a healthy diet.

Quick Tip:

Don't smoke, or quit if you do. Cigarette smoking has many harmful effects on the body, including early and more severe degeneration of the back, which is getting more and more attention. Nicotine—in any form—blocks the transport of oxygen and important nutrients to the spine's discs. Starved of oxygen, the discs are much less able to repair themselves and tend to collapse at a much earlier age than is seen in non-smokers. This painful collapse—degenerative disc disease—can lead to chronic back pain. Moreover, should any surgery be needed, smokers have been found to have 50% slower healing times and a high rate of failure in the healing process.

Summary:

*There are many types of treatment for the lower back but the **main** **emphasis should be on not just removing pain but preventing it and** **supporting the structure of the spine to prevent problems.** Chiropractic care and physical therapy will help with this and should include exercises and rehab care at home. Medications, ice and heat will help through the acute pain, but **rehab is a must**!*

*Before you can heal, there has to be a **good diagnosis for what is the** **underlying problem**. Once you find the cause, you can find the remedy. After all, you already know the affect: pain. In most cases, **back problems** **are the result of many years of improper posture and structural issues** which means there is **never a quick fix**. Even those who end up having to have surgery are facing months if not years of rehab and relearning proper habits for sitting and standing.*

*For less serious problems that do not need surgery, there are a **number of alternative therapies**. However, it is important to know which is appropriate for your needs and your condition. It is also **important to** **know the proper way to employ these therapies or you could likely cause** **more damage overall**.*

6

Diet For A Healthy Back... And A Healthy Body

We Are What We Eat!

WARNING: If you want to eat hamburgers and fries, do not read this section; it will make you too healthy!

Well your back is an indicator of how healthy you are and will respond badly to bad diet and positively to a healthy diet, and what you eat.

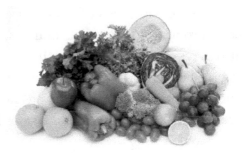

Fresh fruit & vegetables

Your diet—is an important part of keeping your back pain free. You may say: "*How's it possible that what I put in my stomach can stop pain in my back?*" It's very simple.

A lot of people who have back pain also have neck pain, shoulder pain and knee pain even pain all over their bodies, and they are wondering why all of a sudden this happens.

It usually happens to people over the age 40. One reason is perhaps that those joints are injured and they are starting to become arthritic. One of the other main reasons is what people eat. Most people have what is called an inflammatory diet. They eat refined sugars and bad fats—such as burgers, fries and sodas. For example, if you have fast food and you eat French Fries, these saturated fats cause a hormone imbalance that causes a lot of inflammation in your body. Also, improper combinations of acid and alkaline foods cause the body to inflame, creating more back pain than you might have already and speed up arthritis and other degenerative changes to the body.

Here is the proper way to eat.

Wholesome Diet and Nutrition

As most people are well aware, good nutrition and a balanced diet are important components of overall health. What may surprise people with back problems is that diet, nutrition and maintaining a healthy weight also plays a major role in back health—by preventing many problems and injuries. The bones, muscles and other structures in the spine need good nutritional support so that they are strong enough to support the body and perform their other functions. Using the following nutritional guidelines, you can go a long way in supporting your doctor's efforts to improve the muscular, structural and neurological integrity of your back.

Alkaline Producing Diet

One of the most important topics found in nutritional science is the significance of maintaining proper chemical pH for good health and having an alkaline diet! There is a lot of information that supports this assertion. Let's look at some of the key elements of maintaining proper chemical balance and the *underlying secret for capitalizing on this important discovery.*

The Basic Chemistry of pH Balance

In high school chemistry we learned about pH: Neutral pH is 7.0, acids are below 7.0, and alkalines are above 7.0.

In health, we have better long-term health if our body's pH is neutral or slightly alkaline. When we have greater acidity, we have a great risk of developing osteoporosis, weak muscles, heart disease, diabetes, kidney disease and a host of other health problems that directly or indirectly affect the back.

According to many scientists who have researched "chronic low-grade metabolic acidosis," eating a diet that has more alkaline and less acidic food, provides the best support for muscle, bone and nerve integrity. Just what kind of diet is that? It's one that's high in fruits and vegetables. That might not seem like a big surprise, but let's first consider the following then return to this important dietary principle.

Acid-Yielding Foods Deplete Minerals

Most people, including physicians, aren't familiar with balancing acid and alkaline foods or the dangers of acidosis, except in the most extreme situations such as, lactic acidosis from over exercise (lactic acid is produced in the muscles when there is limited oxygen, and causes cramping pains), ketoacidosis (when diabetics start burning their own fat), and renal acidosis (which can be a sign of kidney failure).

When acid-yielding foods lower the body's pH, the kidneys coordinate efforts to buffer that acidity. Bones release calcium and magnesium to re-establish alkalinity, and muscles are broken down to produce ammonia, which is strongly alkaline. By the time the response is all over, your bone minerals and broken down muscle get excreted in urine.

Long term, excess acidity leads to thinner bones and lower muscle mass, kidney dysfunction and related musculoskeletal problems, all of which affect the functional integrity and vitality of the back. These problems can be compounded by normal aging, which can increase acidosis, bone loss and muscle wasting. These factors play essential roles in bone formation. Low magnesium levels can also cause muscle cramps, arrhythmias and anxiety.

The Secret to Maintaining Proper Alkaline pH Levels

It is important to maintain a proper pH chemical balance for the health and vitality of the back. I'll share the underlying secret for maximizing pH balance while minimizing dietary stress. After all, lye, ammonia, milk of magnesia, baking soda and several poisons are high in alkalinity, but you couldn't support a healthy systemic pH with a daily cocktail of these "highly alkalizing" substances.

The secret to maintaining proper alkalinity is eating a diet primarily consisting of fruits, vegetables, nuts and seeds. The addition of grains, meat, dairy and all other foods should be limited as much as possible and be based on your individual requirements, capacities and health goals. Of course, athletes and those enjoying good health may take more liberties than those who are sedentary and/or those experiencing or predisposed to back problems. However, even many athletes experience best results with a whole food plant-based diet.

If you can't do the alkaline diet because it's too hard, then you can cheat by taking green powder from the health food store, known as wheat, or barley or rye and many other grasses usually combined, which has been dehydrated to concentrated forms. You take 1 tablespoon typically in the morning and evening in a glass of water. This will help raise your pH, but the more fruits and veggies and less meats and junk food the better.

What About?

Dairy Products

The strongest evidence to support the benefits of maintaining an acid-alkaline balance relates to osteoporosis. Epidemiological studies demonstrate that Americans consume more calcium-rich dairy foods than almost every other nation, and yet we have the highest rates of osteoporosis. This may sound counter intuitive.

Here is why!

Mother's milk is alkaline, ~7.2 to 7.4 which is neutral and perfect for helping to maintain blood ph of ~7.4. Cow's milk is acidic-6.4 (7 being neutral). Mother's milk being an excellent alkalizing food promotes healthy muscle, bone, sinew and nerve development for infants and children. Cows' milk and related dairy products may be rich in calcium, but dairy foods also produce an acid yield, and the primary reason is the pasteurization of most milk consumed. The acidity it causes helps actually leach calcium out of bones leading to osteoporosis.

Pasteurization, in addition to destroying or altering some important vitamin and mineral contents, also destroys the important enzymes needed to help metabolize and assimilate the calcium and other important minerals. Consider also that cow's milk is optimum for development of physical bulk for baby cows and bulls, but its protein is significantly greater than the protein in mother's milk, producing an acidifying effect for human systems.

Furthermore, dairy consumption increases the risk of kidney stones and kidney failure. Many back related problems can be directly linked to kidney issues. Kidney problems can cause back pain at the sides of the spine just above the hips. Fortunately, there are excellent milk substitutes, such as Rice Dream (Original) and Almond Milk (Plain) that have the look, taste and feel of milk without the problems of dairy consumption.

Soy

Many people have been influenced by the brilliant hype and marketing of soy as an excellent substitute for meat as a source of protein for aspiring vegetarians. There are many studies linking soy to a variety of problems including the presence of large quantities of natural toxins or "anti nutrients" including potent enzyme inhibitors that block the action of trypsin and other enzymes needed for protein digestion. Soy also contains goitrogens—substances that depress thyroid function, which can contribute to weight management problems. Additionally a very large percentage of soy is genetically modified, and it also has one of the highest percentages of contamination by pesticides of any of our foods.

Soybeans are high in phytic acid, present in the bran or hulls of all seeds. It's a substance that in addition to producing an acidifying effect on the system, can block the uptake of essential minerals, calcium, magnesium, copper, iron and zinc in the intestinal tract. Acid washing in aluminum tanks leaches high levels of aluminum into the final product. The resultant curds are spray-dried at high temperatures to produce a high-protein powder. A final process to the original soybean is high-temperature, high-pressure extrusion processing of soy protein isolate to produce textured vegetable protein (TVP).

There are some soy products that are, in fact, good for you—but only certain types and in limited quantities. Fermented soy, which includes natto, miso and tempeh, is a health food for most. But soy formula, soy protein isolate, soy protein concentrate seem to be appearing in a whole variety of so-called "vegetarian" products, which I believe is contributing to much damage to both children and adults in this country, and it should be used sparingly at best because it is acidifying.

Grains

Grains, such as wheat, and corn, have a net acid-yielding effect, regardless of whether they are in the form of white bread, breakfast cereal, pasta or whole grains. Grains tend to be the most frequently consumed plant food in the United States, and account for more than 50% percent of the plant foods eaten by Americans. In addition to their acid yield, grains displace more nutritious fruits and vegetables, and for those with gluten intolerance, can be an additional causal or contributive factor to allergies, gastrointestinal and other inflammatory issues that can directly or indirectly impact back health and vitality.

Gluten intolerance is common due to the vast amount of wheat and corn in our diet. Symptoms include headaches, lethargy and back pain. So limit your grain use, especially wheat and corn, and substitute with oatmeal, rye and other grains if you must.

Processed Foods

All processed foods are acid producing!

Because many of us live in cities far from where food is grown and produced, there are many obvious advantages to food processing, including mass production at cheaper overall costs. Therefore, a large profit potential exists for the manufacturers and suppliers of processed food products. Other benefits of food processing include toxin removal, preservation, easing marketing and distribution tasks, and increasing food consistency. In addition, it increases seasonal availability of many foods, enables transportation of delicate perishable foods across long distances, and makes many kinds of foods safe to eat by de-activating spoilage and pathogenic microorganisms.

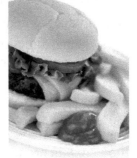

Processed foods are also often less susceptible to early spoilage than fresh foods, and are better suited for long distance transportation from the source to the consumer. Fresh materials, such as fresh produce and raw meats, are more likely to harbor pathogenic microorganisms (e.g. Salmonella) capable of causing serious illnesses.

Stay away from junk food like this

With the benefits of cost, convenience and availability there are also several drawbacks that leave a long list of health consequences. Food processing lowers the nutritional value of foods and introduces hazards not encountered with more natural, unprocessed products.

Processed foods often include food additives, such as flavorings and texture-enhancing agents, which may have little or no nutritive value. Preservatives, such as nitrites or sulphites, added or created during processing to extend the shelf life of commercially available products may cause adverse health effects. Use of low-cost ingredients that mimic the properties of natural ingredients (e.g. cheap chemically-hardened vegetable oils in place of more-expensive natural saturated fats or cold-pressed oils) have been shown to cause severe health problems, but are still in widespread use because of cost concerns and lack of consumer knowledge about the affects of substitute ingredients.

Processed foods include anything that comes in a box, can or bottle. They include a long list of common foods such as breakfast cereals, cookies, cakes, pies, desserts, microwave foods, sugar substitutes (e.g., aspartame, Splenda, Sucralose, Equal), processed oils and even foods touted as excellent protein sources such as soy products.

It is best to avoid all processed food as much as is practical. Most are acid producing and all contribute to compromised functional integrity of all systemic functions, including the health and vitality of the muscles, bones and nerves of the back.

Avoid Hydrogenated and Partially Hydrogenated Oils

The first thing to understand about fats is that the essential fatty acids they contain are truly *essential*. They are the "active ingredient" in every bodily process one can name, including brain cell function and nervous system activity of the spine, hormones and intra-cellular messengers, glandular function and immune system operation, cell wall function and digestive-tract operation. The good news is that the body requires a relatively small percentage of the fats from high quality sources. This is where modern dietary practices have contributed to many problems, including back and bone issues.

Hydrogenation is the process of heating oil and passing hydrogen bubbles through it. The fatty acids in the oil then acquire some of the hydrogen, which makes it denser. If you fully hydrogenate, you create a solid (a fat) out of the oil. But if you stop part way, you create semi-solid *partially hydrogenated oil* that has a consistency like butter, and it's a lot cheaper.

Unlike butter or virgin coconut oil, hydrogenated oils contain high levels of *trans fats*. A trans fat is an otherwise normal fatty acid that has been "transmogrified" by high-heat processing of free oil. The fatty acids can be double-linked, cross-linked, bond-shifted, twisted or messed up in a variety of other ways. In short, trans fats are poisons, just like arsenic or cyanide. They interfere with the metabolic processes of life by taking the place of a natural substance that performs a critical function. In addition to this acidifying affect on the body, trans fats contribute to diseases such as multiple sclerosis, allergies that lead to arthritis, and in the meantime they will make you fat! Trans fats include all hydrogenated, partially hydrogenated mono- and bi- glycosides. They are common constituents of many processed foods that are directly or indirectly contributing to a whole host of modern day back problems.

Flax seed or oil contains the important fatty acids, in particular, omega-3, for ensuring functional support of the myelin sheath which provides outer coverage and support for the spine and central nervous system.

Meat, Fish, Pork and Poultry

Eating large amounts of animal protein, which includes meat, fowl and seafood, releases sulfuric acid through the metabolism of sulfur-containing amino acids which contribute to greater acidity. This acidic shift can be offset with greater consumption of fruits and vegetables (rich in potassium bicarbonate).

Those wanting to optimize the functional integrity of the back should limit the use of all flesh foods. The commercial processing, susceptibility to harboring harmful bacteria, viruses, spoilage, heavy metals, pesticides, antibiotics and growth hormones can also exacerbate both acidity and other challenges to our overall health and vitality. Pork and shellfish can be particularly problematic because they are scavengers and generally are more susceptible to additional toxic loads on the body including PCBs, heavy metals and other bacterial and viral issues. The high uric acid resulting from an animal-based diet contributes to essentially washing out our bone structure.

High Vegetable Based Protein

The best protein source for supporting back, muscle and bone support is from vegetable sources. In 1988, the *American Dietetic Association* noted that the vegetarian diet of sufficient calories is more than adequate to support all of our nutritional needs, including our protein requirements. As a matter of fact, one of the biggest problems with the American diet is too much protein, especially from animal sources.

There are many views and much controversy concerning the relative strengths and weaknesses of the vegetarian versus the meat based diet. Studies show that in the past, ancient diets consisted of a broad range of percentages of animal to plant food ratios from almost exclusively vegetarian to primarily animal based diets with inconclusive evidence of the superiority of either propensity. I believe, however, that for today's purposes the vegetarian diet tends to be superior to the animal based diet for several important considerations that I will list here:

- The vegetarian diet is more likely to promote a more favorable alkaline to acid balance with the advantages of the alkaline foods already noted earlier.

- The vegetarian diet, consisting primarily of fruits and vegetables in their natural, unprocessed state, is higher in the vitamins, minerals and other nutrients needed for healthy bones and structural support.

- Fruits and vegetables are rich in calcium and potassium salts, natural alkaline buffers. In preindustrial society, we ate a larger amount of fresh fruits and vegetables, which have high potassium to sodium ratio. Today, because of heavily salted, processed and fast foods, combined with a low intake of fruits and vegetables, the ratio is significantly lower in favor of sodium. That reversal contributes to a lower pH and our dependency on potassium.

- Commercial animal products today are generally more inclined to contain harmful antibiotics, pesticides, growth hormones and many other environmental toxins in their tissues which are more problematic today than in past preindustrial eras.

- Most Americans tend to both overeat and poorly combine their meat-based meals.

- Animal based foods, which include dairy products, are more likely to harbor bacteria, viruses and other infectious conditions. Animal based diets are also more conducive to contributing to parasites. Both factors can contribute to poor back health.

- Muscle cramps are actually caused primarily by mineral deficiencies; minerals are richer and more bio-absorbable from fruits and vegetables.

- Fruits and vegetables are also susceptible to bacteria, viruses, insects, pesticides and other environmental toxins. However, due to bioaccumulation, the animals that feed on plant-based foods contain several times more of the toxins than the plants they eat.

Acidic Fruits

Although various fruits such as citrus fruits and tomatoes are acidic, they still have a net alkaline yield once their constituents get to the kidneys. This is based in large part on how their vitamin, mineral and other constituents are metabolized with enzymes and related metabolic adaptive and interactive dietary processes.

The bottom line is that the best dietary advice is to emphasize fruits and veggies in the overall diet. Your diet is far more important to overall pH level than supplements alone.

Fruits and veggies are all one needs according to Dr Douglas Graham who wrote the book 80/10/10 because they contain 80% of good carbohydrates, which most of our cell walls in our body are made of, and 10% protein and 10% good fats. We do not need a lot of protein like we are lead to believe and too much is bad.

> *Quick Quiz:*
>
> Which of these are fruits?
>   a. Grapes
>   b. Zucchini
>   c. Cucumber
>   d. Green beans
>   e. All of the above
>
> Answer: All of the above are fruits; they all grow on a vine like a grape. Vegetables, by definition grow as a root or on top of a root like a potato or head of lettuce.

In fact, if your urine contains protein as a waste, you're in trouble. The body does not throw away protein easily. Many world-class athletes were fruitarians and only ate fruit. These were Dave Scott, six time winner of the Ironman Triathlon; Sixto Linares, world record holder in the 24 hour marathon; Paavo Nurmi, holder of 20 world records and nine Olympic medals in distance running; Robert Sweetgall, the world's premier ultra-distance walker; Roy Hilligan, Mr. America bodybuilding champion—Stan Price, world record holder in the bench press—Dan Millman, world champion gymnast - Henry Aaron, all time major league home run champion; and many more.

Dr Jim Sharps, a naturopath and author of *Basic Principals of Total Health,* states there are many factors regarding meat and dairy such as, rampant disease, antibiotics, hormone injections, compromised animal diets, as well as ecological, ethical and moral considerations. A fruit and vegetable based diet promotes total health for you, society, and the planet.

Now, you must eat a pound of fruit a day to get the caloric intake. This is difficult so if you must eat grains, and meat or fish like most of us, then at least eat a diet that is healthy and contains a lot of fruit and veggies, and make sure the meat is organic and devoid of chemicals and hormones.

Alkalizing & Acidic Foods

The charts illustrate some common alkalizing and acidifying foods:

ALKALIZING FOODS		
FRUITS	**VEGETABLES**	**ORIENTAL VEGETABLES**
All Berries	Alfalfa	Daikon
Apple	Asparagus	Dandelion Root
Apricot	Barley Grass	Kombu
Avocado	Beets	Maitake
Banana	Broccoli	Nori
Cantaloupe	Brussels Sprouts	Reishi
Carob	Cabbage	Sea Veggies
Cherries	Carrot	Shitake
Coconut	Cauliflower	Umeboshi
Cranberries	Celery	Wakame
Currants	Chard	**SPICES/SEASONINGS**
Dates	Chlorella	All Herbs
Figs	Collard Greens	Chili Pepper
Fresh Fruit Juice	Corn	Cinnamon
Grapes	Cucumber	Curry
Grapefruit	Dandelions	Ginger
Honeydew Melon	Dulce	Miso
(stand alone)	Edible Flowers	Mustard
Kiwi	Eggplant	Sea Salt
Lemon	Fermented Veggies	Tamari
Lime	Fresh Veggie Juices	**SWEETENERS**
Mangoes	Garlic	Granulated Cane Juice
Nectarine	Green leafy veggies	Honey, Raw
Orange	Horseradish	Molasses
Papaya	Kale	Stevia
Peach	Kohlrabi	**OTHER**
Pear	Lettuce	Apple Cider Vinegar
Pineapple	Mushrooms	Banchi Tea
Raisins	Mustard Greens	Bee Pollen
Tangerine	Okra	Dandelion Tea
Tomato	Onions	Flax
Tropical Fruits	Parsley	Fermented Soy, Organic
Watermelon	Parsnips	

PROTEIN	Peas	Ginseng Tea
Almonds	Peppers	Green Juices
Chestnuts	Potato and Yams	Green Tea
Whey Protein	Pumpkin	Herbal Tea
Powder	Rutabaga	Kombucha
Flax Seeds	Salad Greens	Maple Syrup
Nuts	Spinach	Milk, Organic, Raw
Pumpkin Seeds	Spirulina	Mineral Water
Quinoa	Sprouts	Olives
Sprouted Seeds	Squashes	Organic Milk
Squash Seeds	Watercress	Probiotic Cultures, Raw
Sunflower Seeds	Wheat Grass	
Tofu	Wild Greens	
Yogurt, Raw	Zucchini	

ACIDIFYING FOODS		
ALCOHOL	DAIRY	**NUTS & BUTTERS**
Beer	Butter	Brazil Nuts
Hard Liquor	Butter Milk	Cashews
Spirits	Cheese, Cow	Peanuts
Wine	Cheese, Goat	Peanut Butter
ANIMAL	Cheese, Processed	Pecans
PROTEIN	Cheese, Sheep	Tahini
Beef	Cream Cheese	Walnuts
Carp	Ice Cream	**GRAINS**
Chicken	Margarine	Barley
Clams	Milk, Pasteurized	Bread
Eggs	Sour Cream	Buckwheat
Fish	Yogurt, Pasteurized	Cereal
Lamb	**DRUGS &**	Cornstarch
Lobster	**CHEMICALS**	Macaroni
Mussels	All Chemicals	Noodles
Oyster	Aspirin	Popcorn
Pork	Drugs, Medicinal	Spaghetti
Rabbit	Drugs, Psychedelic	Wheat Germ
Salmon	Drugs, Legal	White Flour
Scallops	Drugs, Illega Flu	Whole Wheat Flour
Shrimp	Shots	

Tuna	Food Additives	**OTHER**
Turkey	Food Coloring	Aspartame
Venison	Herbicides	Bottled Juices
BEANS &	Pesticides	Catsup
LEGUMES	Preservatives	Coffee
Black Beans	Vaccinations	Distilled Vinegar
Chick Peas		Equal
Green Peas	**FATS & OILS**	Mayonnaise
Kidney Beans	Avocado Oil	NutraSweet
Lentils	Canola Oil	Potatoes,
Lima Beans	Corn Oil	Preservatives and Additives
Pinto Beans	Hemp Seed Oil	Processed Foods, All
Red Beans	Flax Oil	Refined Oils
Soy Beans	Hydrogenated Oils	Salad Dressings
Soy Milk	Lard	Salt
Rice Milk	Olive Oil	Splenda
White Beans	Partially	Sucralose
	Hydrogenated Oils	Sugar, All Processed
	Safflower Oil	Sweet N Low
	Sesame Oil	Tea, (except herbal)
	Sunflower Oil	Tobacco, All
		Vinegar
		Water, Tap
		Wheat Germ

Other Important Dietary Considerations

Prescription Drugs As Part of Your Diet

There are obvious benefits to using prescription drugs and careful consideration is required in pursuing alternative herbal and other protocols. However, even in cases where they are providing benefits, it is important to note that all drugs are acid producing and should be avoided as much as practical. Always work with a qualified health professional when considering alternatives to prescription drugs.

A Word on Glucosamine and Chondroitin Sulfate

There is a continuing controversy over the effectiveness of glucosamine and chondroitin sulfate for back pain support. In spite of some brilliant marketing, results are remarkably unimpressive with many of the newer well-designed studies showing little to no effectiveness.

Studies show that glucosamine supplemented with chondroitin can have side effects including nausea, diarrhea, constipation, drowsiness, stomach pain, irregular heartbeats, hair loss and gastrointestinal upsets. Some people suffer from major side effects such as intraocular hypertension where high pressure builds up inside the eyes as a result of using chondroitin.

Because glucosamine is made from shellfish shells, people who are allergic to seafood should use it cautiously, watching for reactions, or avoid it entirely. As for chondroitin, it can cause bleeding in people who have a bleeding disorder or take a blood-thinning drug. Diabetics must also be careful as it might elevate insulin levels in blood. Patients on blood thinners must use chondroitin only after consulting their primary physician. They add nothing to improving the alkaline-acid ratio. In my judgment, the risks tend to outweigh the potential benefits, and therefore are not recommended for back support, health and vitality.

Microwaved Foods

Microwaved foods are subjected to very high temperatures that alter the molecular structure of the food, which robs it of essential nutrients required for good muscle, tissue, bone and nerve development and support.

Proper Food Combining

The digestive system is fundamentally mono-trophic, which means that it works best when we eat one food at a time. Eating large varieties of foods puts a stress on the digestive juices, which can lead to fermentation of carbohydrates and putrefaction of proteins consumed leading to several metabolic disturbances in addition to its acidifying effect on the system. In his book, *The Basic Principles of Total Health*, Dr. Jim Sharps covers the topic of proper food combinations in further detail.

Most people eat foods that are improperly combined. If you eat a hamburger, you are eating proteins and carbohydrates. This is a potential food combination problem. Carbohydrates and proteins do not mix well.

It takes acidic enzymes (HCL stimulates the production of pepsinogen) to break down protein and alkaline enzymes (amylase) to break down carbohydrates. If you eat both, your body does not know what to do and the carbohydrates grow bacteria, which feeds on the proteins and it turns into a big toxic mess. This becomes what is called leaky gut syndrome. The toxins leak into your blood stream and inflame your body.

Try not to eat proteins and carbohydrates together. These are called acid foods and alkaline foods and when eaten together this confuses the digestive system.

I have attached a food-combining chart to help guide you in choosing proper food combinations.

FOOD COMBINING CHART
DO NOT COMBINE FRUIT WITH OTHER FOOD EXCEPT GREEN NON-STACHY VEGETABLE, SEEDS AND MOST NUTS

ACID FRUIT
Blackberries
Grapefruit
Kumquat
Lemon
Lime
Orange
Pineapple
Pomegranate
Raspberries
Strawberries
Tangerines
Tomatoes*
(Eat before other fruits)

GOOD

SUB-ACID FRUIT
Apple   Kiwi
Apricot   Mango
Blueberries   Nectarine
Cherimoya   Papaya
Cherries   Peaches
Fresh Figs   Pears
Grapes   Plums

GOOD

SWEET FRUIT
Bananas
Dates
Dried Fruit
Lychee
Persimmon
Raisins
Prunes

GOOD

MELONS
Cantaloupe
Casaba
Crenshaw
Honeydew
Persian
Watermelon

(Eat them alone or leave them alone)

POOR

*Tomatoes combine best with non-starchy vegetables, nuts, seeds, olives, cucumbers, Avocado, and seed peppers

NON-STARCHY VEGETABLES
Aruguia   Asparagus   Broccoli   Brussels Sprouts
Cabbage   Celery   Chard   Collard
Cucumber** Dandelion   Eggplant   Endive
Escarole   Green Beans Kale   Lettuce
Parsley   Spinach   Sweet Pepper Turnips
Zucchini**

**Eat sparingly: garlic, leeks, onions, radishes, scallions, shallots

EXCELLENT

STARCHY VEGETABLES
Artichokes   Cauliflower
Beets   Corn
Carrots   Pease

**Botanical classified as a fruit, but its biochemical composition places it in a non-fruit food combining category.

Excellent   Excellent   Excellent   Excellent

PROTEINS***
Coconut
Nuts
Olives**
Seeds
(Eat Sparingly: beef, butter, cheese, eggs, fish, fowl, milk, pork, soybeans, yogurt)

Poor

Oily Fruit
Avocado
(An Excellent source of essential fatty acids)

Good

CARBOHYDRATES
Potatoes
Soaked/sprouted beans
Soaked/sprouted grains
Squash**
Yams
(Eat Sparingly: cooked, beans, grains, grain products)

***Proteins also combine poorly with starchy vegetables

Poor

Avoid processed foods, white sugar, white flour, salt, coffee, caffeinated tea, commercial juices, vinegar, strong spices, heated/fried oils, chemical additives and preservatives, and chlorinated and fluoridated water.

Quick Tip:

Good Food Combinations:
- Meals with foods just from one category acid or alkaline.
- Soaked in water nuts or seeds with sub-acid fruits or sweet fruits
- Starches and vegetables
- Proteins and non-starchy or slightly starchy vegetables
- Acid fruit and sub-acid fruit, or sub-acid fruit and sweet fruit

Poor Food Combinations:
- Sweet fruits with acid fruits
- Fruits with vegetables, proteins, starches
- (except celery and pre-soaked nuts and seed)
- Proteins and starches/carbohydrates
- Fats and proteins

Cleansing and Rebuilding Diet

Juicing, fasting, metal elimination, parasite elimination programs, colon, kidney and liver detox programs all contribute to improving the health and vitality of the back.

There are many other herbs and supplements that can be used to help with a variety of issues that directly or indirectly impact overall back health. I want to emphasize the variety of dietary and herbal strategies for supporting back health and vitality.

Parasite Elimination

Parasites are the most powerful species in the world, according to many biologists. They quietly work behind the scenes to take over the body, control it and sometimes are never detected. Worms, bacteria, viruses, amoeba and other species can enter the body many ways such as dust, sneezing, and food. The foods that carry most of the parasites that work quietly behind the scenes are meat and fish. These contain worms, and when these enter the body the whole body can swell over months or years and stay mildly swollen. I recommend that all meat eaters to do a parasitic cleanse for 30 days 2 times a year. There are various ways to do this from fasting to herbs or medication, but I recommend a company called Advanced Naturals for a product called Paramax. It's powerful but safe and easy. Take natural herbal pills for 30 days and only the bad parasites will be eradicated from your body. Go to www.advancednaturals.com for ordering. It's worth doing, especially if you're a meat and fish eater.

When I took these my tongue turned bright green for two weeks and my kids said *"eeyyooo why is your tongue green"*. Well it had something to do with dead parasites exiting. I felt so much better after those 30 days and all of the swelling that I had was gone. I did it again six months later to see if my tongue turned green again but it didn't. I guess they were the results of the parasites exiting. I no longer eat much meat. However one day I did eat a steak that tasted slightly bad and sure enough I had welts all over my body from some form of parasite in the meat that was now in me. I retook the Paramax and it cleared up.

Important Vitamins and Minerals for Back Support

There are several vitamins and minerals that are important in the development and support of back health and vitality. The following is a list of the most important vitamins and minerals:

Vitamin A is an antioxidant that assists the immune system in fighting off diseases. It is good for the back because it helps repair tissue and assists in the formation of bone. It also helps the body use protein effectively. Additionally, the body can convert beta-carotene into vitamin A. Beta-carotene can be found in dark green leafy vegetables such as spinach and in most orange vegetables and fruits such as apricots, nectarines and cantaloupe, carrots and sweet potatoes.

Vitamin B12 is necessary for healthy bone marrow and for the body - and the spine - to grow and function normally. Vitamin B12 can be found in green leafy vegetables, such as spinach, kale and broccoli.

Vitamin C is necessary for the development of collagen, which is an important part of the process that assits cells in the formation of tissue. This is extremely important for healing problems caused by injured tendons, ligaments and vertebral discs, as well as for keeping bones and other tissues strong. Vitamin C can be found in fruits, such as strawberries, kiwi fruit and citrus fruits (e.g. oranges, guavas, grapefruits) and tomatoes, and many vegetables, such as broccoli, spinach, red and green peppers, sweet potatoes and white potatoes.

Vitamin D helps improve calcium absorption, which is important for the development of strong and healthy bones. Adequate calcium absorption is particularly important to help prevent development of osteoporosis, a disorder characterized by weak and brittle bones in the spine that can result in painful vertebral fractures. It also prevents certain cancers. The best source is sunlight-30 minutes a day, and the supplement with D3, when sufficient sunlight is not available. Fish oil and egg yolks also contain vitamin D, but can also contain environmental and other contaminants that may be counterproductive to healthy back support.

Vitamin K is needed for the bones to properly use calcium. The combination of vitamin K and calcium works to help bones throughout the body stay strong and healthy. Vitamin K can be found green leafy vegetables such as spinach, kale and broccoli. It is also a blood coagulator so if your taking blood thinners or prone to strokes and heart attacks avoid taking vitamin K.

Calcium is essential for bone health and helps maintain the necessary level of bone mass throughout the lifespan and especially in old age. Adequate calcium intake is particularly important to help prevent development of osteoporosis, which results in weak and brittle bones in the spine and other bones that can result in painful vertebral fractures. Calcium can be found in dark green leafy vegetables such as spinach, broccoli and kale, peanuts, peas, black beans and baked beans, as well as in a variety of other foods such as sesame seeds, blackstrap molasses and almonds. I included a commentary on calcium supplements at the end of this discussion on vitamins and minerals and a chart of good sources of non-dairy calcium at the end of this chapter.

Iron is needed for cells to remain healthy as it helps them receive oxygen and gets rid of carbon dioxide. It also aids in the production of myoglobin, an important element of healthy muscles, which are needed to support the spine. Excellent sources of iron include lentils, beans, grains and green leafy vegetables such as spinach, kale and broccoli, and dried fruit such as prunes, apricots, figs and dates.

Magnesium is important for the relaxing and contracting of muscles. It also helps maintain muscle tone and bone density, which in turn can help prevent back problems. Further, it assists in the body's absorption of calcium and use of protein. Magnesium can be found in whole grains and whole-grain breads, beans, seeds, nuts, potatoes, avocados, bananas, kiwi fruit and green leafy vegetables such as spinach, kale and broccoli.

While these tend to be the most important vitamins and minerals for back support, a healthy diet will provide the full spectrum of vitamins, minerals and other phytonutrients required for the synergistic absorption and utilization of nutrients required for overall back health and vitality. It's important to note that the best sources for these vitamins and minerals are from a diet rich in a variety of fruits and vegetables. Among the benefits of food based vitamins and minerals are avoidance of possible over dosage occurring from synthetic vitamins/mineral supplementation. Therefore food-based supplementation is a way to ensure proper ratios of vitamins and minerals for best absorption and utilization, and thus contributes to proper systemic alkalinity.

Does Calcium Supplements Help?

Millions of women dutifully take calcium supplements to help maintain their bone mass and reduce their chances of developing spinal atrophy and severe osteoporosis as they age. But do supplements have any real benefit in alkalizing the body?

Some see a benefit from supplements, but there is no clear evidence that supplementation works in the absence of sound dietary practices. Acid-alkaline balance is primarily a food issue. Isolated vitamins and minerals may help in severe deficiencies, but there is no chemist in the world who can formulate the right amounts and right ratios of vitamins and minerals as well as Mother Nature. Proper calcium absorption requires magnesium, boron and other important minerals that are balanced for optimum bio-utilization and provided in whole foods, primarily fresh fruits and vegetables.

Potassium has turned out to be a crucial mineral for maintaining bone. High-potassium diets—that is, those rich in fruits and vegetables—slow bone loss, mainly by promoting alkalinity. All animal products are higher in sodium and phosphorous, which may show well on bone mass and density tests, but the evidence clearly demonstrate that these foods have clearly contributed to higher compromised bone integrity than diets rich in fruits and vegetables. In general, supplements will enrich the financial assets of supplement suppliers more than the health, vitality and integrity of our bones, muscles, joints and nerves, which are important for back health and vitality. A handful of raisins, a couple of dates, a banana and most green vegetables each provide rich supplies of bioavailable potassium, calcium, magnesium and other phytonutrients that support back and spinal integrity.

If you take supplements, opt for the citrate form, such as calcium citrate and magnesium citrate. Fumarate, aspartate, and succinate forms of minerals also have an alkalizing effect. My biggest caution is in the use of calcium carbonate, which though highly absorbable is generally sourced from dolomite, which also contains lead and other heavy metals that can affect the central nervous system, joints and contribute to other conditions that can have primary or secondary effects on the back.

Some supplements, such as coral calcium, have been promoted as a way to restore alkaline PH. Coral calcium is also largely calcium carbonate, which contains heavy metals that can accumulate in the joints and muscles, as well as affect the central nervous system, all of which are important to support health and vitality. It's also not as well absorbed as the citrate form.

> **Did You Know?**
> The typical American diet relies on products for over 70% of it's calcium. But YES we can get enough and better absorbable calcium without dairy products!

Non-Dairy Sources of Calcium

Approximate calcium content per 8 oz. (1 cup):

Food Source	Mg.	Food Source	Mg.
Cow milk	300	Sea Vegetables	
Buffalo milk	600	Wakame, reconstructed	3,500
Goat milk	320	Kombu, reconstructed	2,100
		Nori, reconstructed	1,200
Collard greens	300	Agar-Agar, reconstructed	1,000
Spinach	275	Dulse	560
Turnip greens	230	Kelp	560
Bok Choy	200		
Kale	150	Other Sources	
Broccoli	150	Cooked Soybean	450
		Tofu	400
Almonds	750	Bean sprouts	320
Hazelnuts	450	Garbanzos	150
Walnuts	280	Black beans	135
Sesame seeds	2,100		
Hulled sunflower seeds	260	Dried figs (10)	270

Chestnuts	600	Orange juice	210
Nut Butters	100	Salmon	490
		Sardines	300
Sesame	425		
Almond	270		
Hazelnut	195	Black strap molasses, 3 tbsp.	470
Sunflower	125	Herbs	Vary
Peanut	35	Grains	Vary

Herbs for Back Pain

There are a variety of excellent herbs than can be used in a strategy for improving back health and vitality. Remember, many components in powerful prescription drugs are herbal extracts. The following are common herbs used to help relieve back issues. These include **anti-inflammatory** herbs (angelica, boswella, bromelain, cat's claw, licorice, rosemary, saw palmetto berries, valerian root), **antispasmodic** herbs (chamomile, cramp bark), **circulation** herbs (bilberry, grape seed extract, gingko biloba), **diuretic** herbs (uva ursi, juniper berries, buchu root) and pain relief herbs (cayenne (topically), feverfew, ginger, kava, mint (topically), stinging nettle, white willow bark). These and additional herbs work well individually or synergistically to address a broad variety of back related issues. Be sure to work with a qualified professional when considering using herbs to ensure best results.

Sufficient Water

Our body is 70 to 75 percent water. An alkalizing diet is a high water content diet, which ensures a sufficient supply to support the many metabolic adaptive and interactive processes to ensure spinal support and functionality. A general rule of thumb is one half your body weights in ounces of water. This number should be adjusted up or down, based on activity level, health and type of diet. The formula is based on 128-pound woman at rest, which translates to 64 ounces or the much quoted 8 glasses a day. A high water content diet consisting of primarily fruits and vegetables (which are more than 70% water) requires fewer additional glasses of water to satisfy the formula than a dehydrating diet consisting of meat, dairy and other dehydrating elements, like alcohol and caffeine.

Snack Ideas

- Fresh vegetables with veggie based and nut butter dips
- Trail mix of nuts, seeds with raisins and other dried fruits
- Smoothie with nut or seed milk with bananas, peaches and/or dried fruit
- Herbal teas—yellow dock, dandelion, nettle, raspberry, valerian root, sage, etc

> *Quick Tip:*
>
> **Proper Snack Combos:**
> - Fruits combine well with celery, lettuce, nuts and seeds (particularly presoaked).
> - Tomatoes and avocados combine with vegetables.
> - Melons should only be combined with other melons.
> - It is better not to combine a grain, starch and a protein in one meal.

Summary:

What you eat will determine your health and the health of your back. An anti-inflammatory diet works best, along with an alkaline diet. Eating mostly fruits and vegetables will give you a whole new lease on health and a pain free back.

A proper diet makes tissues heal faster and reduces inflammation. Eating food in the proper combination where one does not mix acid and alkaline foods will go a long way to digesting food properly and reducing inflammation in the body. **You are what you eat, so let's eat right.** *Stay away from fast foods, refined sugars and flour, and meat and potato diets.* **Drinking plain water is also crucial for it rehydrates the body and discs and flushes out toxins.** *Everything else is diuretic and reduces the body's rehydration. So eat fruits and vegetables mostly raw, and drink four to six eight-ounce glasses of water a day and see the results.*

7
Putting It All Together

Five Simple Steps to a Healthy, Pain Free Life
Posture Is The New Sexy

If you want to look taller and more confident and appear to be in great physical shape even if you have a belly, then having good posture will do this. Having your head tall, shoulders back, forward pelvis, legs and knees straight is sexy. Posture also burns calories – improper standing or sitting does not.

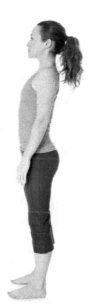

Having a belly does not stop good posture. It can even help it by causing the pelvis to shift forward, which helps contain the discs in the back from bulging. I had a patient in my office, Sharon T., who was 75 lbs over weight and 6'0 tall. But she commanded respect, looked like an athlete and was beautiful because she walked tall with perfect posture.

So here's how you have good posture:

Good posture

How to Stand

- Stand with your heels six inches apart, toes and knees slightly facing outward.

- The knees are not locked but are straight or pointed slightly out.

- Pelvis is forward, let the belly drop but don't sway backward.

- Imagine you feel a string pull you up from the top of the head.

- Relax the chest and don't try to stick the chest out.

- Lower your chin slightly extending the neck.

- Practice this until you feel very little muscle being used and relaxed.

- Have someone take your picture to show you your posture.

- If you're having a hard time, tape a three-foot stick to your buttocks and your upper back and it should be vertical. Practice walking with this taped to your back until you get how it should feel.

How to Bend and Lift

- Bend at the hips and knees, not the back.

- Keep the knees aimed outward toward the little toe.

- Keep a backward small arch in your back so it acts like a basin, not a hill.

- Point your sits bones or ischia out behind you .

- Your legs are shoulder width apart.

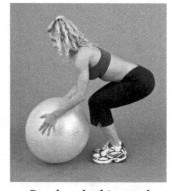

Bend at the hips and knees not the back

- To lift, just straighten the hips and knees at the same time, always keeping a backward arch in your back or a basin in your lower spine.

> *Quick Tip:*
> Use this bending procedure when sitting down in a chair as well.

> *Quick Tip:*
>
> When lifting something bulky where you can't bend at your hip (such as putting groceries in the trunk of a car) then you want to pivot forward on one hip while the other leg balances straight out backwards behind you and place the items down.

How to Lift an Object

So many people make this mistake! We forget to check our body mechanics while lifting, yet too much of this type of movement can be very damaging to your back.

When lifting, follow these steps:

- Get close to the object. Bend your hips and knees and grasp the object firmly, keep the back straight or better yet arched slightly backward. Lift straight up (don't twist!) in one fluid motion. Hold the object close to your body.
- Move close to where you want to place the object.
- Bend your knees when lowering the object.

> *Quick Tip:*
>
> Never twist your back. If you need to turn, move the feet to turn. Twisting tears the discs in your back or injures the muscle or ligament in the back.

How to Sit

There are at least three main ways to sit properly.

1. Chair
2. On the floor cross-legged
3. Squatting

In all three ways, you use the same mechanics:

- Establish a solid base, but use a wedge under your sits or butt bones with the fatter end of the wedge at the back.
- Relax your belly where the center of gravity sits.
- Open up your mid back by relaxing your chest.
- Roll one and then the other shoulder three times and let it settle down and back to neutral.
- Tilt neck very slightly forward.
- Relax your belly and chest down.
- Roll your shoulders back and let them relax.
- Pull your head and neck back so it sits on your shoulder and drop the chin slightly.
- By the end of the process, if you feel any muscle not relaxed, relax these but make sure your good posture is still held as in these photos.

How to sit in a chair

- Make sure you have a solid seat, and if needed try a wedge in the back of the chair.
- Use the arm rests if you have them or put arms at the base of the seat and slowly drop your backside into the back of the chair.
- Relax the mid back into the back of the chair, and if there is no back, relax the belly and chest. Roll shoulders backward three times and let them settle back down.

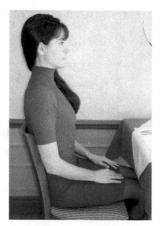

The correct way to sit in a chair

- Pull your head and neck back to neutral and drop the chin slightly so the head rests slightly forward on the shoulder. Imagine a spring pulling up from the back of your head.

By the end of the process, if you feel any muscle not relaxed, relax these but make sure your good posture is still held as in these photos.

Quick Tips:

Try alternating other ways to sit for a few minutes to give your constant posture a break.

a. **My favorite way to sit**-Scoot up to the edge of the chair or stool and put my legs well under it . This makes you want to fall forward so to compensate you lean back and you automatically sit upright with a gentle arch in my back and shoulders back and down and tilt the pelvis forward. I like this way because you don't need to think about it, it's automatic proper posture. If you can sit this way 60% of the day of actual sitting that would be great.

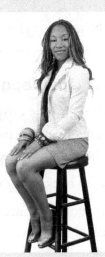

Best way to sit

Or you can use a kneeling Swedish chair, which does the same thing, for part of the day.

b. Slump, yes I said slump. It's okay for 5-10 minutes. It allows the muscle to relax and opens up the low back joint spaces.

c. Try sitting on an exercise ball for part of the day. They even make these with back supports now. But get it fitted so your knees are bent at a 90-degree angle, no more, no less.

> *Quick Tip:*
>
> When using a computer keyboard make sure that when you are sitting in a chair the proper way, the keyboard is well within arm's reach where the arms are not reaching! The arms should be relaxed where the elbows are directly below the shoulders, which are back and down.
>
> The monitor should be at eye height.

How to sit cross-legged

- Sit with legs crossed on the floor on a cushion under the sit or ischial bones with pelvis shifted forward.

- Keep back upright and straight.

- If your hips are too tight then put a rolled up towel or pillow under each knee.

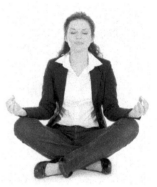

Sitting cross-legged position

> **Did You Know?**
>
> Squatting is the hardest position for most westerners. In developing countries, this is how they sit for hours. It places tension in the right direction, thus increasing range of motion in the hips, knees, ankles and allows more flexibility while maintaining a neutral spinal posture.

How to Squat (which is how you're supposed to "sit" in nature because it opens up or promotes great joint motion and prevents arthritis in your hips, knees and lower back joints)

- Bend at the knees (using a chair beside you for support if you need to) and bring buttocks to the heels as close as possible. Heels should be flat, if not, stretch the back of the legs daily.

- You should have the feeling being back a little where the knees are over the ankles but not ahead of them much.

- Knees should be pointed 45 degrees out.

- The back should have an arch in it.

- If you hold a yardstick from the upper back to the lower back it should lie flat.

- If you need more support, rest your back against a wall as you are squatting.

- If this is hard then start with one minute and add time as the days go on so in the end you can squat for 10-20 minutes or longer at a time.

- You can do a partial squat and come down as far as your knees and hips allow using a chair beside you as support until you no longer need that support.

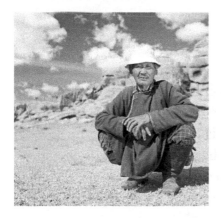

Squatting position is seen all over underdeveloped countries. Squatting position helps keep the entire lower body flexible.

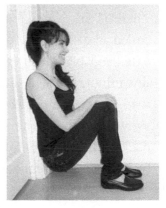

Alternate squatting position for those who have trouble squatting

How to Sleep

There are 3 ways to sleep:

1. *The supine or on your back position:* This is sleeping on your back. This is a good position because it relaxes the back by relaxing the arch in the lower back.

2. *The side lying position:* This sleeping position should be held without twisting the lower back.

3. *The prone or on your stomach position*: This is sleeping on your stomach. Although this position is not recommended by most doctors, I am not totally opposed to it. It forces your back into extension, and it usually requires your neck to be rotated for breathing. So, it increases the range of motion, or the mobility, of the neck and the spine. This reduces scar tissues and arthritis. Be aware that despite its benefits this can also be a risky position because it can cause pinching of nerves due to increased pressure on the joints.

> *Quick Tip:*
>
> There is an exercise used in physical therapy and Pilates called the McKenzie exercise. It puts the spine into extension or makes the patient lie in prone position for a few minutes. This exercise program is designed for people who have diminished C-curve of the lower back. This shows that the prone position is not a total no-no for low back pain. It definitely has its benefits; however, it should be held with a great degree of caution.

How to sleep in supine position or on your back:

- Use two soft pillows. One should be halfway stacked on the other. Make sure that the edge of the bottom pillow is positioned under your shoulder blades and the top edge of the pillow on top is under your shoulders.

- Rotate shoulder down and away from the neck.

- Feel the spine lengthen and relax.

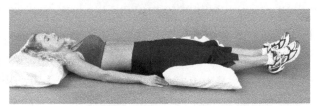

*One correct way to sleep in supine
position or on your back*

> ### *Quick Tip:*
>
> Use a cervical pillow, which has a thicker base and a hollow center to fit the curve in your neck. This is only to be used if you have a significant curve in your neck or a very rigid neck. These pillows can be beneficial for the neck, but they can also cause kinking of the spinal nerves, and put excessive compression forces on the cervical facet and uncinate joints, which causes neck pain. So try it but be cautious.

> ### *Quick Tip:*
>
> Putting a pillow under the knees while lying on your back can help take the pressure off the back and lengthen it.

How to sleep on your side

- Lie on your side with one or two pillows under your head.

- Push with your upper hand down on the bed or floor and scoot your pelvis or pubic bone back several inches, flexing your knees.

- Set your knees at around 120 degrees to the body, not too straight, not too bent, but half way in between.

- Pull your pillow forward toward your knees until you feel your back lengthen to relax.

- Keep your knees together to prevent the low back from twisting

- An alternate way is to put 2 thick pillows on both of your body by the knees and when you lie on one side the top knee goes on that pillow, and when you rotate to the other side the other top knee goes on that pillow (see below).

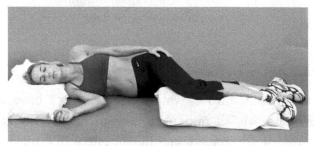

How to sleep on your side with top knee on the pillow

Quick Tips:

Three ways to position your arm

1. Place your bottom arm along side your body, in front of you.

2. Placed under the pillow and head but not rotated on the elbow with your palm up as that will cause much strain on your medial elbow and cause tendon strain otherwise known as the golfer's elbow. Golfer's elbow is the inflammation of the medial epicondyle, which is a bony prominence in the inside of our elbow. It usually involves strain of the muscles or tendons attached to that area.

3. Placed behind you, slightly rotated forward. Use this position when you have shoulder pain because it will ease tension in the shoulder.

> **Quick Tip:**
>
> Use a pillow to support your knees and to prevent twisting. There are three ways:
>
> 4. Place a pillow between your knees.
>
> 5. Place one in front of your knees.
>
> 6. If you flip from side to side, you may lose the pillow accidentally as you roll in your sleep. Before you sleep set one pillow on both of your sides so when you roll to either side, your knee will always have a pillow on which to rest.

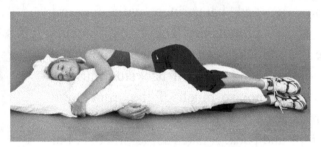

How to use a body pillow for
better support for the lower back

Proper Walking/Running Posture

Can you believe that we in the Western world walk and run incorrectly? In developing countries, they walk by pushing off rather than stepping forward. I call this gliding. In the urbanized west, we over flex our hips and overuse our hip flexors or psoas and quadriceps muscles as we walk,

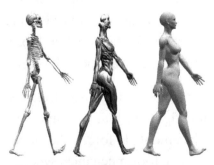

Picture of walking the right way

causing tightness and undue pressure on the knees, hips and back, which in turn causes arthritis.

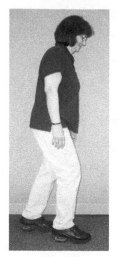

See the forward flexion, bend at the waist and shortening of the hip and bent knee and forward body tilt .She is using the front of the thigh-quadriceps and psoas hip flexors more.

See the opening of the hip, straighter knees, standing up straight of body in greater extension and she is using the back of the thighs- hamstrings and gluts more.

Wrong way to walk

Walking is about gliding using the gluteals or buttocks and hamstrings with forward propulsion. The body remains stable while the buttocks, legs and feet are doing the action. So you are using push off backside muscles to propel you and not so much of the front thigh quadriceps muscles. Try it; it's very different and very easy on the hips and back. It takes some practice, but after a while it's easy and will become the norm. It will make you feel like your gliding.

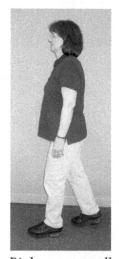

This gliding strengthens the buttocks or gluteal muscles, which support pelvic anteversion or good

Right way to walk

healthy posture. This also prevents forward falls, and in geriatrics it prevents fractures of the hip, which can lead eventually to death due to immobility—a blood clot formation or pneumonia and possible death.

This gliding also stretches to the psoas muscles, which are already too tight on many people, and helps restore the proper anterior pelvic placement. It forces the upper torso to be upright and taller. It allows proper foot mechanics where your heel strikes first and the rest of your outer foot lands, keeping a better arch in your foot.

It allows the hip to hang during the swing phase, stretching the hip muscles and relaxing the hip and knee joint. It also allows soft landing so no damage occurs to the hip or knee joint, but does allow enough pressure during the landing phase to prevent osteoporosis. It provides more free blood flow and supply, helping prevent varicose veins and clots.

Are these enough reasons to learn how to walk properly? I believe so.

> **Quick Tip:**
>
> You know you're walking right when you feel yourself coming off your back foot big toe, and feel the back thigh muscles and buttocks working.

So here's how you do it:

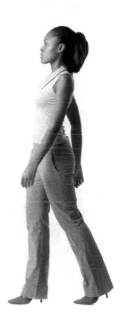

- Start off shifting your weight to the left leg while bowing slightly at the hips and lean forward.

- As you move forward by straightening your left leg, your right leg bends at the hip and the knee.

- As your hips and weight move forward, extend the right leg while tightening the left Gluteal muscle (butt muscle) as it pushes the heel into the ground.

- Aim the knees toward the same side little toe.

- Place the right foot, heel first on the ground, knees slightly bent.

- Relax the left leg.

- Repeat on the other side.

Walking Step-by-Step

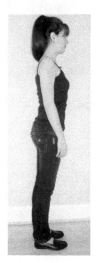 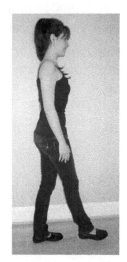 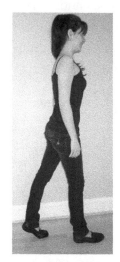

Walking step-by-step (1)   *Walking step-by-step–*   *Walking step-by-step-heel*
glide right leg, contract   *strike right foot and relax*
gluts and hamstring rear   *left gluts and hamstrings*
left muscles (2)   *and get ready to glide left*
leg now (3)

Quick Tip:

The gluteals or buttocks do the work rather than the front hip, thigh quadriceps and the psoas/hip flexors. So it feels that the muscles in the rear, and not the front, are doing much of the work more and this indicates that you're doing it right. You butt will look good if you do this. So practice, practice, practice! It will take some relearning, but with all the benefits and a great butt workout, isn't it worth it?

Running:

Same as walking, but you need to feel it in the hamstrings and gluts and keep upright.

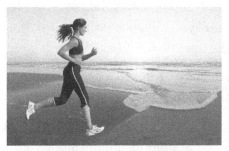

Right way of running, standing up straight using hamstrings/glutes

Diet: What You Eat Will Improve Your Health

A proper diet will reduce your inflammation and let you heal quickly and prevent degenerative changes. In other words you are what you eat- "live" food such as fruits and veggies make you alive, dead foods such as burgers and fries will kill you faster, but will first cause disease that weakens

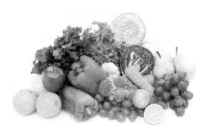

Fresh fruits and vegetables

your muscle, bones, joints and speeds up arthritis, disc bulges, scar tissue- which leads to pain.

To summarize, let me leave you seven important dietary considerations for supporting optimum muscular, bone, spinal and overall back health and vitality:

1. Eat primarily whole foods, consisting primarily of fresh, raw fruits and vegetables. The best way to eat is to get a blender and blend up fruits and veggies in the morning equivalent to 5-7 bananas. Fruit and veggies are 90% water so that's good, but you need to eat a lot to get your daily 2,000 to 3,000 calories depending on your size.

2. Avoid all processed and refined foods as much as possible.

3. Avoid dairy, hydrogenated oils, preservatives, additives (especially MSG), flavorings and substitute sugars as much as possible.

4. Use whole food supplements, i.e., selected foods, herbs and super foods such as royal jelly, bee pollen, acai, noni and other nutrient-dense and therapeutic food-based supplements.

5. Restrict grain and soy products consumption, based on individual requirements and capacities.

6. If meat is eaten, it should be eaten sparingly with vegetables only, and it should be antibiotic and hormone free as much as possible.

7. Learn and apply the basics of proper food combining to minimize acid production and optimize assimilation of important nutrients.

8. Take green powder of different grasses -one tablespoon two times a day of green powder (wheat grass, alfalfa sprouts, spirulina are examples) from the health food store to alkalinize your body if you don't eat enough fruit and vegetables.

9. Take at least 1,000 IU a day of vitamin D3 if you get less than 20 minutes a day of sun.

A healthy diet calls for many vitamins, minerals, other important plant-based nutrients, and a number of healthy choices that can be directly beneficial for helping back patients. While the above is not designed to be an exhaustive dissertation on dietary considerations, I have tried to provide some very important principles and information for equipping and empowering you to make better choices for optimizing back health and vitality.

The Mental Game—Think Positive!

Your thoughts are important and they will either help or hurt you. My patient Mary S. was depressed and all doom and gloom about her back. She said, "I'm never getting better", so I said,

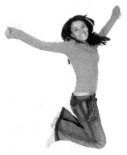

Think positive

"Well then you probably won't." She looked at me and said, "Why would you say that?" I said, "Because you're convinced you won't get better and what you concentrate on grows." It is true, so why not concentrate or visualize you getting better or of you feeling better. Even if you have trouble believing keep telling yourself, visualizing you're getting better. Then you will.

> **Quick Tip:**
> Watching a funny TV comedy while exercising, breathing hard, increasing the heart rate is up on say a stationary bike for 15-30 minutes in the morning starts the day off right. It really gets you in a good mood and you will have natural hormone endorphins released into your body, which are the feel good ones that reduce pain. It works and is my personal favorite tip.

If you ever read the book "The Secret" by *Rhonda Byrne* or any books on Laws of Attraction such as "The Key" by *Joe Vitale*, they talk about how what you concentrate on can become your reality. So thinking about your back pain only makes it worse. Easy for me to say as I don't have back pain, but once I did from an injury. I can tell you by saying to myself "I feel good", "I feel good" over and over even if I didn't always believe it did reprogram my brain to feel better.

Stress has been found to make an already existing back problem worse. Meditation helps with this, Relaxing in a quiet room lying down or sitting with proper posture for 30 minutes a day will help with this immensely. Exercise such as aerobics or lifting weights 30 minutes 3-4 times a week, helps alleviate stress.

Exercise: Stretching, Strengthening and Proprioception

Three types of exercise are needed for the back to recover.

1. Stretching exercises to increase flexibility

2. Strengthening key muscles that support the spine

3. Proprioception or balance that allows proper nerve communication from the brain to the joints and muscles, brings back equal firing of both sides of the muscle to the back.

Stretching

Stretching key tight muscles will relieve joint space tightness. The key muscles to stretch are the hamstrings, psoas hip flexor muscles, and gluteal and piriformis muscles. Strengthening key muscles creates stability for the spine and proper alignment.

Keys to stretching:

- Stretch to just prior to pain-don't overstretch

- Use continuous stretch and don't bounce or jerk

- Stretch for 15-30 seconds

- Breath through it-it helps relax and get oxygen to the muscles

---

Did You Know?
Beginning at age 30, the human body loses around half a pound of muscle every year.

Scary isn't it? This muscle loss is directly responsible for hip fractures and falls, later in life. Moreover, nearly half the people who break their hip don't survive it too long after.

The muscles burn the most calories, so if you don't have muscles, your body is prone to fat and flab. Remember, fewer muscles = more fat in the body!

Weight Lifting—Not Sure If It Is For Me!

Weight lifting isn't for everyone; it's easy to hurt yourself, and can be rather hard on your joints, not totally necessary for toning your body. Stretching is the way to go. Research has shown that you can build and tone your muscles by stretching. It's true, and a new study proves so.

"Stretching appears to do more than just increase range of motion," says study author *Arnold Nelson*, an associate professor of kinesiology at Louisiana State University in Baton Rouge. *"The extent to which some people improved was surprising,"* he says. *"Some people had fantastic improvements."*

> *Quick Tip:*
>
> The key muscles to stretch are:
>
> - Back of thigh or hamstrings
> - Buttocks or gluteal muscles & piriformis muscle
> - Front of hip flexors or psoas muscle
> - Long back muscles that run up and down the side of your back bone, including the multifidi muscles

Strengthening

Spineless is a term used for folks who show weakness. So get a backbone and start an exercise program to strengthen your back. Do this three or four times a week. Exercise helps produce natural pain killer hormones called endorphins and makes you feel great naturally. A strong back gives support and prevents injury and pain. Building muscle is about building it for endurance, not for bulk. It's about getting muscle strong enough to do many chores throughout the day, such as holding groceries while walking to the car. The key muscles to strengthen are the abdominal, gluteal-buttocks, and multifidi muscles.

Keys to Strengthening:

- Stretch lightly before strengthening.

- Do one to three sets of 15 repetitions.

- Use 25%-50% of maximum weight.

- On the last set hold it for five to ten seconds.

- Don't push through the pain. Don't over strain.

- Mix it with aerobics to get the lungs and heart rate going to for 15-30 minutes such as swimming or cycling, which are two great exercises. With swimming you can hang on the edge of the wall and kick, or just run in the water or paddle until you can feel like you can swim.

Proprioception or Balance

Prorioception is a medical word for balance as it pertains to the brain communicating with the rest of the body but mostly to the smaller muscles of the back. When you balance on a wobble board, for example, you can feel the small muscles of the back firing. These are the multifidi muscles, which help the vertebrae, stay aligned. Of course there are many other muscles in the body that need to be flexible, strong and balanced.

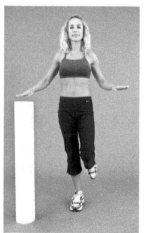

Keys to Proprioception:

- Stand on one leg on the floor, eyes open for one minute twice daily, switch legs.

- In the second week, close ones eyes and do the same.

Proprioception is balance

- In the third week use a wobble board (Go to www.DrDabbs.com for this) and stand on this eyes open for two to three minutes daily.

- After the fourth week stand on the wobble board and do three sets of 10 shallow knee bends while trying to maintain balance for two to three minutes daily.

Dabbs Accelerated Back Care System

Doing a system of rehab exercises is crucial in keeping the body finely tuned to keep up with the day to day stresses we place on it. The system of exercises and day-to-day activities we do must be done with good posture and form, and this will help maintain or rebuild better posture, which is the key to a healthy spine.

I developed the "Dabbs Accelerated Back Care System", which has all the tips and exercises in succession on DVDs so you can do them every day or every other day for six weeks. You do these for 15-20 minutes **with me** in the leisure of your own home to become healthy. Visit me at www. DrDabbs.com and get free tips and don't miss the Dabbs Accelerated Back Care System tab or www.DrDabbs.com/Product where you can purchase all the equipment including exercise balls, wobble boards, foam rollers, elastic bands, and the system itself. This was developed over the last 23 years of practice by interviewing MDs, chiropractors, physical therapists, physical trainers and putting it to the test with patients over 22 years. It works!

If you are in acute pain and can't do exercises, then lie in the recovery position where you're on the floor on your back. Put your feet and legs on a chair at 90-degree angle. Lie there for 20-30 minutes. This really takes the pressure off the back.

Activities of Daily Living: Putting it All Together in Your Daily Life

So every day is a new day, and a day when you can improve your back, your posture, and your health. It's never too late and with just a few days of practice, it will all change for the better. Your daily routine should involve practice, practice, practice of good posture and exercises to improve your posture this is how it should look. I call it the,

Dr. Dabbs Daily Back Care Routine

Use post-it notes as reminders—on or all around your home and work reminding you about proper posture.

Morning in bed: Wake up and stretch. You need to stretch the muscles and joints out before placing weight on them. Grab your knees and pull them up to the chest and hold for 30 seconds, then lay them flat and tighten the abdominals and gluts 10 times in a row for two to three seconds each time. Roll over on your hands and knees and sit on your heels and reach as far forward as you can. Hold that position for 20 – 30 seconds. Stand up from bed and arch backwards putting your hands on your back as you arch. Squeeze your shoulder blades back too.

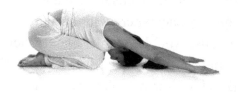
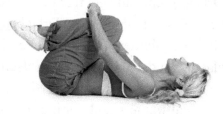

Stretching—cat stretch   *Stretching—pull your knees to chest*

In the shower: While the heat is on your back, squat down so your buttocks are close to your heels. Don't squat on your toes or forefoot, this puts too much strain on your knees, but rather place the weight on your heels when squatting. Your knees are pointed 45 degrees (slightly-half way) out and away from each other. Sit like this for 30 seconds to five minutes with the heat on your back. Then stand up and arch backward for five to ten seconds.

To dry off, dry one foot at a time by pulling up one foot and balancing on the other. Then grab two ends of the towel behind you and stretch your arms backward and away from each other and pull the shoulder blades together. Then put the towel around one foot and pull it back stretching

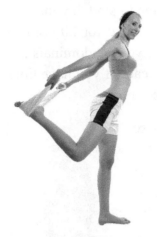

the front thigh while balancing for 15 seconds then try the other foot. Also stretch the neck in all directions.

Brushing your teeth: Brushing your teeth or washing your face in the morning can be challenging on the lower back after getting out of bed. When at the sink, bend by hinging forward at the hips (NOT the back) while keeping the back arched backward or held straight as you bend at the knees.

Good hip and back stretch when toweling off

Getting dressed: Do three more squats before getting dressed and hold each position for 20 seconds each. When putting clothes on, if you have to lift one leg, do it standing and slowly so you balance on each foot for 20 seconds. When putting on a shirt, reach back into the sleeves and squeeze the shoulder blades together.

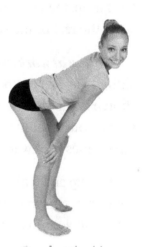

During breakfast: Eat breakfast, drink your coffee while standing, or sit on an imaginary chair with your back resting against a wall holding you up. Read the paper this way. Do a few more squats.

Bend at the hips, knees not the back when at the sink

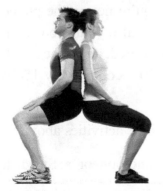

Practice sitting in an imaginary chair against a wall or your partner

Driving: To get in, back into your seat, sit down with your legs outside the car still, then turn with your whole body and bring your legs into the car. Make sure you have a good support pillow in your car and make sure your car seat does not allow you to slump. Your pelvis should be forward with a slight arch in your low back.

At a stop light or if stuck in traffic, use this time to stretch your neck side to side, back to front and tuck your chin backward for 20 seconds each time. Lift your leg up and down and tighten your abdominals and buttocks individually and in succession of 10 reps each if you have time. This helps activate the core muscles to stabilize the spine.

Parking: When parking at work, park far away so you can walk, using proper walking technique so that you are gliding using your buttocks and hamstrings for each step. See Chapter 8 for this. If your workplace is on a higher floor of the building, take the steps. If it's too far up, then take the elevator part way and take the steps the rest of the way.

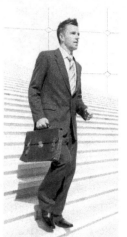

Sitting at work: See how to sit in Chapter 7. While sitting, do the buttock and abdominal contractions, stretch your neck all directions every 30 minutes. Keep your shoulders back and roll your shoulders three times backward every time you sit in your chair.

Walk steps, park far away and walk — it's good for your health

Get up and walk as much as possible. Squat every hour or two if you can. If you have the space then try sitting on your imaginary chair with your back on the wall holding you up for as long as possible while reading or on the phone.

A headset may be good for the neck, but if you're not on the phone all day, you can hold the receiver to your ear and raise your elbows up and down slowly as an exercise. Switch ears when tired. Arch back with your neck and lower back sitting or standing for 10 seconds every 15-30 minutes.

Set reminders every 30 minutes to do any of these activities above.

Sitting on an exercise ball that you can bounce on or a Swedish kneeling chair works well for part or all day sitting.

Manual labor or grocery shopping: If you're active during the day in your job and not sitting all day, then exercise by lifting the groceries with your arms, bending at the hips and knees, not the back. Hold your arms outstretched from your body sideways for exercises. Take rests in between by lowering the arms. Squat whenever you have a chance to look for and grab items from the floor or lower shelves. Always keep your back arched slightly backward or straight and don't lock your knees back.

Sports, gardening, and exercises: All of these are good to do if you keep a good posture, so keep active. Stretch before and after the event. Squat or bend at the hips and knees when gardening if possible, or kneel on a soft mat. Or just do counter squats where you are sitting in an imaginary chair at a counter, or squatting and getting up, or walking 25 minutes a day works. Exercise at the gym, but do not lift weights that are too heavy. If you can do three sets of 15-20 reps then it's not too heavy.

Once you're home and relaxing: If at night you're relaxing watching T.V. or reading a book, don't sit on a couch or in bed that forces you lower back into flexion. Get up and walk around, squat on the floor while watching and do your daily stretches—see Chapter 7 for this.

Back to Bed: When your day ends, be happy with your accomplishments for the day. Be grateful and say out loud everything you did right for the day, not just about what you read here. Relax the mind and meditate, keeping out all negative thoughts so your muscles and mind can relax.

Summary:

To have a healthy back one must learn to:

1. **Have proper posture** *while standing, sitting, sleeping, walking and running*

2. *Have a **good diet***

3. *Have a **good mental attitude** in life*

4. **Incorporate key stretches, strengthening and proprioception exercises** *three to five times a week.*

5. *Do a regimen **of daily activities to support the back** and keep it in the best shape possible.*

6. *Meditate or do aerobic exercises 30 minutes a day 3-4 times a week to reduce stress*

8

No Surgery, No Meds

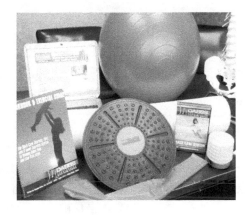

The Dabbs Accelerated Back System

I have been involved in treating more than 10,000 patients in my office with back pain and less than one percent of these patients knew what to do for their own backs. They rely on me, and their medical doctor for help. They have to make multiple visits to my office and many other offices such as physical therapy, neurosurgeons, and psychiatrists and get many expensive, sometimes painful tests. They lose time from work, and sometimes they lose pay or even lose their job. They lose out on life with their family and loved ones, get angry or depressed, even commit suicide as my patient Jared did, or die overdosing on prescription meds as my patient David did.

So I wanted to creat a system that can be taken home for **less than a price of one doctor visit,** or one test. I wanted a system that **saves time** from lost work and from spending it at Doctor's waiting room. I wanted to give you a system to help reduce or eliminate and prevent your back pain so **you can enjoy your lives** and your family's lives again.

So I invented the **Dabbs Accelerated Back Care System**. It is a complete system with all the low-tech equipment such as:

- **5 instructional DVD**
- **Wobble board**
- **Exercise ball**
- **Foam roller**
- **Elastic band**
- **A manual book**

This is where you get all the tips you need for back care and three levels of exercises; you do each level for two weeks and by the end of the sixth week you should feel a lot better. It's based on three levels of exercises:

- Beginners (level 1)
- Intermediate (level 2)
- Advanced (level 3)

People of any age group from 7-90 can do these.

How It Works

It works by concentrating on proper posture, balancing muscles, increasing flexibility and strength in key muscles that are involved in back pain .You must do this in a certain order and use proper form so as to not reinjure your back. Exercising without a system and without guidance may have no results or worsen the condition.

What It Does

It will take you on an adventure with me where you will watch and participate with me, physical therapist, Joanne Colburn, and sports trainer, Tiffany Hayden. You will be doing the exercises daily or every other day for 15-20 minutes starting with level 1 beginners for two weeks, then progressing to level 2 intermediate for two weeks, and finally reaching level 3 advanced for two or more weeks. I will be doing these with you step by step, creating a more balanced body, a stronger more flexible spine and working the mind to feel better. It does it with the best forms of care mentioned in this book like the best of stretching, strengthening key muscles and proprioception or balance, massage, positive thinking, diet, yoga, pilates etc etc… It this comes with the kit. I guarantee this will work in 60 days or your money back. You have my word on that.

Seven Reasons You Must Try Dabbs Accelerated Back Care System

1. Save on cost and time
2. Equips you with easy-to-use tools to rehabilitate your own back
3. One of a kind effective system developed through research
4. Developed by a group of leading and innovative professionals
5. Satisfaction guaranteed
6. Helps to avoid surgery and other painful procedures
7. Gives you back the quality of life you deserve

TRY NOW.

To learn more of the basics of back care, we're going to teach you good posture, more tips and exercises, but it is best demonstrated on videos. Visit www.DrDabbs.com and fill out the web page to get the **free** video "**Back Pain 101**" and also get your **free EBook: 15 Tips for Back Pain** .You can even have a **personal consult** with me and my office. So visit www.DrDabbs.com for this. Your back and health deserve it.

Or email me at DABBSBACKCARE@VERIZON.NET. It is always a pleasure to have me assist in your road to recovery from back pain. *I am here to serve you.* Again, please visit www.DrDabbs.com and receive several priceless BONUSES.

✓ NEW Free Relief Guide - 15 Tips To Back Pain Relief

✓ DVD - Back Pain 101

✓ FREE Newsletter- FEELING GOOD AGAIN!

✓ FREE one-on-one consult with me, Dr. Dabbs

As mentioned earlier in this book, I spent years and years of research and travel in my pursuit of finding a cure for back pain. Now, it's my time to assist others.

My purpose is to "educate, inform and heal" people. I feel truly blessed with the knowledge I've gained and feel so thrilled to spread the word through seminars, workshops, discussions—both online and offline.

Thank you for reading this book. I hope you learned a lot, more importantly, it my sincere hope that you spread the word around. Encourage your friends and family to read this book, so that they too can be enlightened to heal their back and body and keep themselves well.

Here's to your good health and success,

Dr. Vaughan Dabbs

Testimonials For The Dabbs Accelerated Back Care System

*Name: Kevin Glover Occupation: Former NFL football player for Detroit Lions	"Doing proper rehab exercises and stretches will keep your back in good shape and the Dabbs Accelerated Back Care System uses the exact exercises involving strength, proprioception and flexibility to reduce your back pain. This system works."
*Name: Jan Jacubik Age: 61 Occupation: Advertising	"I had surgery for lower back pain and the surgeons said they needed to do more surgery because I still had pain. However, upon doing the Dabbs Accelerated Back Care System for six weeks, I now am virtually pain-free and can avoid future surgery."

*Name: Donna & Don Cook Age: 58 & 57 Guidance Counselor and Teacher	"Before using the Dabbs Accelerated Back Care System, drugs were making us groggy and we felt like we were not enjoying life. A very short time after using the Dabbs Accelerated Back Care System, we feel great and we now feel we can live a normal life without pain. The system gives you all the tools and it saved us thousands of dollars in doctor's bills and saved us time in multiple trips to the doctor's office. "
*Name: Karen Kurtz Age: 51 Occupation: Administrator	"Before, I could not sit at all and had severe lower back pain and could not enjoy my family. Now after using the Dabbs Accelerated Back Care System, I can once again sit and enjoy my family and it feels great."
Name: Laura Henry Age: 27 Occupation: Administrator	"After having months of severe lower back pain, I am now 100% pain-free, thanks to Dabbs Accelerated Back Care System."
Name: Mary Siegel Age: 55 Occupation: Administrator	"Using the Dabbs Accelerated Back Care System, in just a few short weeks, I had complete relief of my back pain."

Name: Donald Jackson Age: 46 Occupation: Administrator	"Before I had back pain and I could not play any sports or do any activities for months, but now after the Dabbs Accelerated Back Care System I can play soccer, golf, softball, baseball, all 99% pain-free."
Name: Candice Cotton Age: 41 Occupation: Social Worker	"Now that I am using the Dabbs Accelerated Back Care System, I have a good night's sleep. I can do all my chores. I can drive with no pain for the first time in years."
Name: Eve Lamb Age 56 Occupation: Financial Analyst	"I haven't felt this good in years using the Dabbs Accelerated Back System."
Name: Moria Allen Age: 50 Occupation: Administrator	"Using the Dabbs Accelerated Back Care System, I find it to be a life-changing experience because now things that were very difficult to do before are now easy again. It's the little things in life that I missed and I have my life back now."

Name: Gordon Travloar Age: 52 Occupation: Accountant	"Before the Dabbs Accelerated Back Care System, I had many surgeries and fusions to the lower back and felt I was reaching a life of disability. After using the Dabbs Accelerated Back Care System, I now have the function and the confidence that I will not be handicapped for the rest of my life, and can carry on to do things that before would have prevented or impeded me."
Name: Jim Gary Age: 73 Occupation: Retired	"I am 73 years old and I am playing softball again, now that my lower back is pain-free thanks to the Dabbs Accelerated Back Care System."

**Dabbs Accelerated
Back Care System**
7910 Woodscape Drive
Clarksville, MD 21029
Call 410-660-7491
http://www.drdabbs.com

Let us thank you with a gift certificate!

Thank you for reading this book.

Come join me for a FREE one-day Intensive workshop:

Why Your Back Hurts

Register today at
http://www.drdabbs.com

G I F T   C E R T I F I C A T E | $1995.00

To: _Our fabulous customer, "YOU" and one complimentary guest_

In the amount of: _One Thousand Nine Hundred and Ninety-Five----------_

One-Day Intensive Workshop - "Why Your Back Hurts"

Redeem today. One gift certificate per person.

Email:
Dabbsbackcare@verizon.net

Share The Health

"The greatest wealth is health" ~**Virgil**

Indeed, it couldn't have been said any better. Your health is your biggest wealth. That is what this book teaches you in so many different ways. You are challenged to take a good look at the way you do things, your habits, your thoughts, the way you treat your back and body, and so much more.

Health is one of the most important components in a person's life; it can also be the number one cause of your downfall. If you don't have good health, you don't have anything. Once you reognize this—work, money and everything else will fall into place.

With this book my goal is to help you raise your level of consciousness. I want you to be aware of your health, and the health of the people around you.

Realize the essence of a transformation is not just about you. It's about the entire world—the people around you. As each person raises his or her level of health consciousness, the world raises its consciousness—moving from unhealthy and dissatisfied to healthy and happy. If you want to see the world as a healthy place, start with yourself first. You'll realize your full potential, and achieve success.

I ask you to share this message of good health with others. It's important that you convey the message of this book to others—your friends, family and associates. Offer them the gift of health. Not only will they become mindful of their health, they, in turn, will raise health consciousness amongst others and help you on your journey.

Make it a commitment to spread the word to as many people as you can. Think about it as a life-saving gift. I believe we can do it, one back at a time.

Additionally, it would be amazing if they could join me on my one-day intensive workshop. You will learn the inside scoop as to why your back hurts and what you can do about it. You will also learn how to put this book into practice, and find out the root cause of your back problem, and what you can do about it. This workshop was specifically designed for you, so sign up at www.DrDabbs.com today.

Remember, it's an opportunity of a lifetime—it's an intensive workshop that is hands on with me as your doctor for the day. It doesn't get any better that this!

I look forward to seeing you soon.

Thank you

About the Author

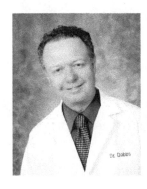

Dr. Dabbs received his Bachelor of Science Degree in Biochemistry from McMaster University in Ontario, Canada in 1982, and his Doctorate of Chiropractic Cum Laude from Logan College of Chiropractic in 1987. In 1990 he received his Diplomat of Chiropractic Orthopedics from Texas Chiropractic College. He went on to start and run one of the most successful Rehab Centers in the USA which is located in Columbia Maryland.

Dr. Dabbs helped start and effectively manage the Spine and Rehab of America of which he was an active board member. Spine and Rehab of America was a public company consisting of 35 clinics across the USA.

Dr Dabbs background includes over 60,000 hours of instruction, rehabilitation, adapted physical education, sports medicine, training, prevention programs. He is a member of the Maryland Chiropractic Association and American Chiropractic Association. He was the first Chiropractor on the Columbia Medical Plan HMO, the largest local HMO in Maryland at the time where he saw the worst of the worst back care patients. 90% were improved with his care. His office has been voted as **"Best Chiropractic office in Howard County in 2011" by Howard County Magazine.**

Dr Dabbs has also been published in top Orthopedic and Rehab Journals and continues to do active research.

A well known speaker and educator, Dr. Dabbs lectures across the country at leading sports medicine clinics, medical offices, medical seminars, and medical conventions.

The dynamic Dr. Dabbs is currently Director of Rehab Center of MD LLC and developer of the nationally based Dabbs Accelerated Back Care System, which is an easy to do for all, home based rehab care system for low back pain found at www.DrDabbs.com. He can be reached at for questions or comment at DabbsBackCare@verizon.net.

Dr Vaughan Dabbs
8600 Snowden River Pkwy ste 101 Columbia MD 21029
tel: 410-720-5555

Email: DabbsBackCare@verizon.net

website www.ThisIsWhyYourBackHurts.com

Developer of "The Dabbs Accelerated Back Care System" 2010
www.DrDabbs.com

Owner of the large Dabbs Rehab Center of MD for 24 years
& Voted "Best Chiropractor Of Howard County 2011"
by Howard Magazine www.DabbsRehab.com

Publisher is numerous Medical and rehab Journals

Speaker and Educator

Board Member and Developer of Spine and Rehab
of America with 35 clinics in 1999-2002

Bibliography

Bar K.P., AL. (2005). *Lumbar Stabilizations: Core Concepts and Current Literature. Part 1*. American Journal of Physical Medicine and Rehabiliation, 84:473-80.

Bond, Mary. (1993*). Balancing Your Body*. Rochester, Vt: Healing Arts Press.

Brill, Pegg. (2001). *The Core Program*. New York: Bantam Books.

Chaiamnuay P, Daramwan J, Muirden KD, et al. (1988). *Epidemiology of rheumatic disease in rural Thailand: a WHO-ILAR COPCORD Study*. Journal of Rheumatology, 25:7.

Darmawan J, Valkenburg HA, Muirden KD, et al. (1992). Epidemiology of rheumatic diseases in rural and urban populations in Indonesia: World Health Organization International League Against Rheumatism COPCORD study, stage 1, phase 2. Annals of Rheumatic Diseases, 51:525-28.

Darmawan J, Valkenburg HA, Muirden KD, et al. (1995). The prevalence of soft tissue rheumatism. A WHO-ILAR COPCORD study. Rheumatology International. 15:21-24.

Dart, Raymond. "Voluntary Musculature in the Human Body: The Double Spiral Arrangement." *The British Journal of Physical Medicine* 13 (1950): 265-68.

Deyo RA, Phillips WR. (1996). Low back pain. A primary care challenge. 21(24): 2826-32.

Dimon, Theodore. Jr. Ed.D (2011). The Body in Motion: Its Evolution and Design. California: North Atlantic Books.

Dixon RA, Thompson JS. (1993). Base-line Village health profiles in E.Y.N rural health programme area of northeast Nigeria. African Journal of Medical Science. 22; 75-80.

Donkin, Scott. (1986). *Sitting on the Job*. Boston: Houghton Mifflin Company.

Ebenbichler G.R, al. (2001). *Sensory Motor Control of Lower Back Pain: Implications for Rehabiliation.* Med Sci Sports Exercise, 33(11): 1889-98.

Fahrni, WH. Conservative treatment of lumbar disc degeneration: our primary responsibility.

Fahrni, W. Harry and Trueman, Gordon E (1965): *Comparative Radiological Study of the Spines of a Primitive Population with North Americans and Northern Europeans.* The Journal of Bone and Joint Surgery, 47-B(3): 552.

Fullenlove, T.M, and Willaims, AJ. (1957). *Comparative Roentgen Findings in Symptomatic and Asymptomatic Back.* Radiology, 68, 572.

Gokhale, Esther. (2008). *8 Steps to a Pain-Free Back. China: Quality Books, Inc.*

Hodges, P.W. (2003). *Core Stability Exercises and Chronic Lower Back Pain.* Orthopedic Clinical N AM, 43: 245-54.

Heliovaara M. (1989). *Risk factors for low back pain and sciatica. Annals of Medicine.* 21(4): 257-64.

Hurwitz E, al. *Treatment of Back Pain: Noninvasive Interventions Result of Bone and Joint Decades.* 2000-2010 Task Force on Spinal Pain and Associated Disorders. Spine 2008; 33: S123-52.

Hutchinson, Alex. *The Globe and Mail.* November 12, 2010. Take a pass on the Advil—swelling may help you heal.

http://m.theglobeandmail.com/life/health/alex-hutchinson/take-a-pass-on-the-advil-swelling-may-help-you-heal/article1808598/?service=mobile

Jackson, RP, McManus AC. *Radiographic analysis of sagittal plane alignment and balance in standing volunteers and patients with low back pain matched for age,and sex.* A prospective controlled clinical study. Spine 1994; 19(14): 1611-18.

Karp, J. (2007). *Muscle Fiber Types and Training.*

Lebouef-Yde DC. (2000). *Body weight and low back pain: A systematic literature review of 56 journal articles reporting on 65 epidemiologic studies.* 25(2): 226.

Lehrich JR, Katz JM, Sheon RP. *Approach to the diagnosis and evaluation of low back pain in adults.* Uptodate.com, April 2006.

Liebenson C. (2007). *Rehab of the Spine: A Practitioners Manual,* 2nd ed. Baltimore: Lippincott, Williams and Wilkins. 612-62.

Luoto, S.B, Heliovaara M.M., Hurii II.M., al. (1995). *Static Back Endurance and a Risk of Lower Back Pain.* Clinical Biomechanics, 1995; 10: 323-4.

Luo X, Petrobon R, Sun SX, Liu GG, et al. (2004). *Estimates and patterns of direct health care expenditures among individuals with back pain in the United States.* 29(1): 79-86.

MacGregor AJ, Andrew T, Sambrook PN et al. *Structural phychological and genetic influences on low back and neck pain: a study of adult female twins.* Arthritis Care and Research. 51(2): 160-7.

Mayer J, Mooney V, Dagenais S. (2008). *Evidence Informed Management of Chronic Lower Back Pain with Lumbar Extension Strengthening Exercises*. 8: 96-113.

McGill, S. (2004). *Ultimate Back Fitness and Performance*. Waterloo, Canada: Wabuno Publisher.

McGill. (2002). *Lower Back Disorder Evidence Based Prvention and Rehabiliation*. 130-1. Waterloo, Canada: Wabuno Publisher.

Osborne and, Cool, J. (2007). *Global Muscle Stabilization Training – Isotonic Protocols; Liebenson*, C, Ed: Rehabilitation of the Spine, A Practinoer's Manual Second Edition Baltimore; Lippincott, Williams and Wilkins. (667-87).

Position yourself to stay well: The right body alignment can help you avoid falls and prevent muscle and joint pain. Consumer Reports on Health; February 2006;8-9.

Posture and back health: Paying attention to posture can help you look and feel better. Harvard Women's Health Watch; August 2005: 6-5.

Polus, B.I, *Muscle Spindle and Spinal Proprioception. Haldeman S*, Ed: Principles and Practice of Chiropractic Third Edition. New York; McGraw Hill: 249-88

Porter, Kathleen. (2006). *Ageless Spine, Lasting Health: The Open Secret to Pain-Free Living and Comfortable Aging.* Texas: Synergy Books.

Punnet L, Pruss-Ustun A, Nelson DI, et al. (2005). *Estimating the global burden of back pain attrituable to combined occupational exposures*. American Journal of Industrial Medicine.

Osborne N, Op Cit. Bernard J, Bard R, Pujol A., al. *Muscle Assesment in Healthy Teenagers, Comparison With Teenagers Lower Back Pain*, Ann Re-adapt Med Phys, 51(4): 263-83.

Sarno, John E. (2010). *Healing Back Pain: The Mind-Body Connection.* Mass Market Paperback

Sharps, Jim. Dr. (2006). *Basic Principles of Total Health. Columbia*

Stenson, Jacqueline. February 19, 2009. *Stretching may offer extended benefits.* http://www.msnbc.msn.com/id/21489011/39285850

Suni J, al. *Control of the Lumbar Neutral Zone Decreases Lower Back Pain and Improves Self-Evaluated Work Ability: A Twelve Month Randomized Control Study,* Spine 2006; 31: E611-20.

Wigley RD, Zhange NZ, Zeng QY et al. (1994). *Rheumatic diseases in China: ILAR-China study comparing the prevalence of rheumatic symptoms in northern and southern rural populations.* J Rheumatol. 21(8): 1480-90.

Yinen, J.J., al. (2006). *Effects of Neck Pain Muscle Training One Year Following Chronic Pain Journal Strength Condition,* and Revs, 20:6-20.

Printed in the USA
CPSIA information can be obtained
at www.ICGtesting.com
JSHW012052140824
68134JS00035B/3398